THE LITTLE DREAM DICTIONARY

THE LITTLE DREAM DICTIONARY

An A–Z Guide to Decoding Your Dreams

Tim Rayborn

MANDALA

San Rafael Los Angeles London

"We are such stuff as
dreams are made on,
and our little life is
rounded with a sleep."

—*The Tempest*, Act IV, Scene 1

CONTENTS

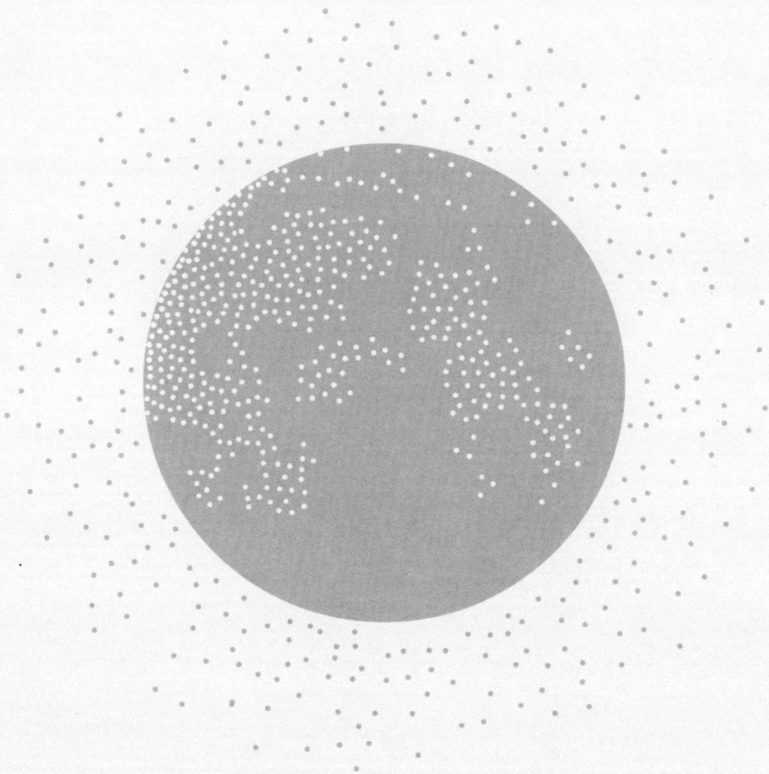

INTRODUCTION

DREAMS HAVE FASCINATED US FOR AS LONG AS WE'VE BEEN SLEEPING AND DREAMING. FROM THE ANCIENT WORLD TO THE MODERN DAY, WE HAVE TRIED TO ANALYZE AND UNDERSTAND WHAT OUR STRANGE NOCTURNAL VISIONS MIGHT MEAN.

Do they give us insights into ourselves? Do they predict future events? Are they messages from an unknown, mysterious beyond? Dreams can be absurd and surreal, and while some are stimulating, even pleasant, others are terrifying.

Why do we dream at all? There are various theories. One says that we dream to help process and catalog memories, while another suggests that dreaming might be an adaptation to keep our visual cortexes healthy in the dark. Dreaming might also help us "rehearse" for the next day.

In any case, the history of dream study and interpretation is long and immense, and varies widely from culture to culture.

Among aboriginal peoples in Australia, many believe that their ancestors dreamed existence into being during a period called the Dreamtime. This age continues to exist in its own reality, and the aboriginal people can visit the Dreamtime in their own night dreams, and perhaps speak with the ancestors.

In ancient Egypt, many people believed that dreams and dream figures were communications from a spirit dimension that was a realm between those of the living and the dead. Such a magical place could bring important communications, including news about the future.

Many seers and prophets would pray to the gods and other entities for visions in their dreams, in order to help guide others and perhaps give tantalizing glimpses into what was to come.

In contrast, some ancient Chinese scholars and physicians held that dreams revealed information about a person's health or mental state.

Even in these earlier times, there were attempts to view dreams in a more detailed way. In the second century CE, Artemidorus, a famed dream interpreter, wrote his *Oneirocritica*, a work devoted to dreams and their meanings. Collected in multiple volumes, it discusses all kinds of topics related to dreams, from human anatomy to the natural world, to how dreams can be understood, as well as the methods and techniques for interpreting them. He stresses that one needs to know about the dreamer (their status, health, background, and so on) in order to properly understand and decipher their dreams.

Throughout the Middle Ages and into the Renaissance, dreams continued to fascinate and beguile everyone from the mightiest monarch to the humblest of farmers. Hieronymus Bosch's famed (and bizarre) painting, "The Garden of Earthly Delights," lays open a fantastical dream world in all of its weirdness, interweaving outlandish images with religious themes. Twentieth-century Surrealist artists would mine their dreams for some of the same richness for their own paintings.

At the beginning of the twentieth century, Sigmund Freud published his landmark book, *The Interpretation of Dreams*, a work that changed how scientists viewed dreams, their origins, and what they are telling us. He maintained that dreams are secretive (trying to hide things), and derive from the unconscious; they are usually a kind of wish fulfillment. All dreams have a connection to something that happened to the dreamer, most often earlier in the day, though the dream content and imagery might come from several different places, such as experiences or memories. Dreams can even be influenced by outside sources while the person is sleeping; you might experience your alarm clock in a dream, for example, as your mind and body try to ignore it and keep on sleeping (a situation that a lot of people can probably relate to!).

Of course, given Freud's work, many have assumed that all Freudian views on dreams have a sexual aspect to them, though he denied this was the case. The phrase "sometimes a cigar is just a cigar" is often attributed to him. And while there's no actual evidence that he said this, the idea applies well to dream interpretation.

Freud's pupil, Karl Jung, explored dreams in his own unique way. Rejecting Freud's theories, Jung maintained that dreams were revealing and mythic in nature, and drew from a shared human experience. They help us to integrate aspects of our conscious and unconscious minds, what he called individuation. Each dreamer can tap into these energies to create a personal myth, to help them integrate and become more whole.

Behavioral psychologist Calvin Hall believed that dreams were almost like performances in the mind's own theater, and that they revealed how we imagine and conceive of our lives. By studying them, we can learn much about ourselves. We can see them as maps for why we choose to do what we do.

Dream studies and interpretations continue today, with many different theories and approaches to working with these mysterious nighttime visitors to our minds.

Of course, researchers have identified several different types of dreams. Here are just a few:

- **Daydreams.** These are flights of fancy that we all indulge in, where our minds wander off. They're not "true" dreams, of course, but they show the power of our imaginations, even when we're awake.
- **Lucid dreams.** These dreams occur in the time between being awake and fully asleep and are often hyper-realistic. The dreamer can even have control over what happens.
- **Nightmares.** The classic bad dreams of childhood and beyond. "Nightmare," by the way, has nothing to do with a horse. The word "mare" comes from medieval English and means a kind of evil spirit.
- **Recurring dreams.** We might dream about being in the same place or doing the same action over and over. Usually, these dreams are trying to tell us something . . . but what?

Ultimately, dreams can mean many different things, depending on whose research you're following. Dreams are often symbolic, with what you see and hear representing something else.

This dictionary offers brief introductions to 1,000 dreams and dream types, to help give you a clearer understanding of what's happening in your mind while you sleep.

It's important to keep a dream journal (like *The Little Dream Journal*), and to write down your dreams and any impressions you felt about them as soon as you wake up; otherwise, you will likely forget them as the day progresses. Don't worry too much about trying to analyze them right away; just write them down! You can revisit them later.

Obviously, this book can only scratch the surface, and these entries represent just some of the more common dream interpretations. Other resources might interpret the same dream differently, and your own personal, cultural, and psychological background will also affect what your dream might mean. Your situation could be quite different, or the entry you are looking for isn't here, simply due to space. If you want to learn more and truly explore the world of dreams and their meanings, see the "Further Reading" list at the end of the book.

You might find that you can combine different entries here to get a bigger picture of your dream's meaning. Let's say, for example, you dream about driving a car, so you look that up. But what color was the car? You can look up color meanings. Do you remember what clothes you wore? Was a friend or relative with you? What was the weather like? Were there trees or houses? Each of these topics has its own entry, and you might find that you can enrich your understanding of your dream by combining several meanings.

Importantly, if you are suffering from sleep apnea, nightmares, sleep paralysis, or possible repressed trauma that manifests in your dreams, this little book can only give you a few insights. You should always seek the help of a qualified professional for medical and psychological concerns.

The world of dreams is endlessly fascinating. Let this little guide be your first step into an amazing journey!

DREAM DICTIONARY

A

AIRPLANE

A dream of being on or seeing an airplane could represent new beginnings in your life or a desire for greater freedom and adventure.

ALARM

Hearing an alarm might indicate that you are worried about a situation or relationship, and you might need to take quick and decisive action to fix it.

ALIENS

If your dream involves aliens, you may be fearful of your future and unknown outcomes. Alternatively, you may be feeling isolated and like an outsider yourself.

ANGER

If you are angry in a dream, it almost certainly means that you're angry in waking life, or are suppressing something that angers you. You need to address it.

ANNOYANCE

If you are annoyed about something in a dream, you might fear that others are working against you in your waking life, or that they are deliberately trying to irritate you.

ANXIETY

To have anxiety in a dream can indicate that you are bottling up emotions and feelings of some kind: fear, anger, resentment. These need a safe outlet.

APPOINTMENT

You may have a real appointment coming up that you are anticipating and possibly feeling nervous about. More generally, the dream could reflect anxiety about your responsibilities and daily schedule.

ARCH

If you pass under an arch in your dream, you are moving toward new opportunities and positive changes, possibly surrounded by those who support you.

AWKWARDNESS

If you are awkward, you probably feel out of place or perhaps judged by someone in your life. Think about ways you could ease this feeling.

AUTUMN

A dream of autumn indicates facing the ending of one cycle and the start of another, or that a harvest of something is at hand, based on your efforts.

B

BEER

Having a beer in your dream can indicate feeling relaxed, that you can take the time to enjoy a break. It might also reflect how you feel about others and your social life.

BEGGING

Begging in a dream will probably have one of two meanings, depending on who is doing the begging:

Someone else is begging you: You probably have a generous nature, especially if you are helping someone in need, and you will probably succeed in your efforts.

You are begging someone else: You might feel that you don't deserve something, or perhaps your insecurities are getting the best of you.

BETRAYAL

Feelings of betrayal can often suggest that you are suspicious of something or someone in your waking life, and you fear that things might not work out.

BICYCLE

Riding a bike is a pleasure for most people, but its dream meanings can be a mixture of different things:

Bicycle color: The color of a bicycle might have specific meanings for you. What was the color of your bike as a child? See also "Colors" for more information.

Riding a bicycle: You probably want or need to maintain more balance in the different areas of your life. Navigating life can be like biking on an obstacle course!

Riding a bicycle with others: You are possibly working with others on some project, or you are striving to be a better partner or friend.

Seeing a bicycle: Your mind might be telling you that you need to take more breaks and enjoy yourself. Remember how fun riding a bike was as a child?

Struggling on a bicycle: If you can't ride your bike well, you might be experiencing self-doubt, and fear that you are not up to some task.

BIRDS

Our feathered friends of all kinds can make frequent appearances in our dreams. Here are some of the more common birds you may encounter in your dreams:

Birds: Seeing birds in general can be telling you something about your dreams, your hopes, and aspirations, and your desire to "fly" freely in life. Birds can also represent harmony and balance in your life, especially if they are singing or chirping.

Birds hatching: If you dream about a bird hatching from an egg, it suggests that new beginnings and new opportunities are on their way, or that you are anticipating them.

Bird's nest: A bird's nest is its home and this dream might be suggesting that you are focused on your own home and security, such as your "nest egg."

Canary: A canary is often a sign that you are happy in a new relationship, or that you would like to be happy with someone new.

Chicken: You might be afraid of something, or you might think that others are gossiping about you behind your back. Or, maybe you're the one gossiping . . .

Crow: There might be something about yourself that is dark or unpleasant, such as a behavior, a belief, or even a bad habit. What do you need to examine and change?

Dead bird(s): One or more dead birds can be pointing to something that has disappointed you, or that you are worried about, perhaps too much for your own good.

Dove: Doves represent peace, love, and harmony, and this dream might be a reflection of you having those things in your life, or your desire to have them.

Duck: Dreaming about a duck might indicate your ability to be flexible, or of having a multitude of talents and skills to bring to the table.

Eagle: Eagles symbolize power, strength, nobility, and courage. This dream might be speaking to your leadership abilities, or your need to cultivate them. Alternately, an eagle can also suggest that you will have to fight for what is rightfully yours, and that you will have the needed strengths to do so.

Falcon: To dream of a falcon suggests that you know what you want and you know what you have to do to achieve it, like a bird hunting its prey.

Flamingo: These funny birds might be trying to tell you that you are overly concerned about appearances (your own or others), even if others accept you.

Goose: You might be on a "wild goose chase" for something that won't happen, or isn't worth your time. There might be a better way of approaching the issue.

Hawk: You might need to focus your "hawk eye" on your surroundings, as there could be trouble, or even danger. Keep watch and protect yourself.

Hen: You might fear that others are gossiping about you or picking on you. Alternately, make sure you are not the one doing the gossiping, because no good can come from it.

Hummingbird: Though you are only one person, your ideas might be much greater than you realize. But be careful to follow through with promises to others.

Ostrich: Are you "burying your head in the sand" and refusing to face up to reality? What situation or person are you trying to avoid, hoping they will just go away?

Owl: Owls represent wisdom and insight, and a connection to your unconscious. Pay attention to what your mind is trying to say to you at this time. Alternately, the owl might symbolize that you are hanging onto something that no longer serves its purpose for you, and it's time to let it go and move on.

Owl's hoot: To hear a hooting owl in a dream can be a bad sign, often indicating disappointment, endings, even death. What is coming to an end for you?

Parrot: Someone might be trying to contact you, but whether this information is useful or just idle chat and gossip is for you to determine, as is if you share it.

Peacock: You can rightly talk about your achievements, but be careful of becoming too boastful and vain. A lot of eyes are watching you.

Penguin: You might need to cool off a bit and not overthink some problem. It's probably not as bad as you think. Find your inner balance.

Pigeon: Pigeons are often associated with messages, but they can also mean that you need to be careful about accepting blame for something that someone else did.

Raven: There might be a death imminent, but it is almost certainly symbolic. Something in your life is dying or transforming, and things will be better for you in the end.

Robin: Robins are usually good signs in dreams, denoting fresh starts and the possibility of new growth and new opportunities, which will inspire you.

Rooster: You or someone you know is being a show-off in your life, and you should probably tone it down a bit, lest you come across as arrogant.

Seagull: You might want to fly away from your problems, to "head out to sea" and be free, but obviously, you'll need to deal with them.

Sparrow: Consider if you are taking on too many burdens. Let others share some of the load, though be careful not to abuse their kindness.

Stork: Storks are, of course, associated with babies, and if you aren't expecting, this dream might indicate a birth of some kind, such as a new idea, a business, etc.

Swan: You could need to be careful about pre-judging someone or something; they could turn out to be far more attractive to you than you first thought.

Turkey: You might be acting in ways that seem foolish or off to others. Perhaps you are not looking at a situation in the best way. Rethink your behavior.

Vulture: You might need to step back and learn a little more, using past experiences. Alternately, someone could be using you, taking advantage of you.

BODY PARTS

Any part of the body can be the subject of a dream, and their meanings are many and varied:

Abdomen: A dream about your abdomen might indicate a feeling that you need to take better care of your health, or that you feel you are, in fact, doing so.

Arm: An arm dream often points to your ability to care for others (such as to hug them), or the issues and challenges you might face when trying to.

Arm (broken or injured): You might feel helpless, restricted, unable to take action, or you could be facing a loss of freedom in some area of your life.

Arms (multiple): Seeing more than two arms (whether on yourself or another) can indicate that you are open to new ideas and opportunities in life.

Armpits: Dreaming of an armpit can offer clues about how you react toward others in social and work situations, and what you choose to reveal about yourself.

Back: To dream about your back might indicate that you are trying to avoid something, or that you need to distance yourself from a situation and rethink it.

Bones: Seeing bones in a dream can mean that you feel unprotected and vulnerable. You might be looking for ways to protect yourself or others around you. Bones may also indicate that there is something in your life that you need to leave behind, whether you like it or not.

Bones (buried): Unearthed bones might mean that something is about to be revealed to you, or you think it will. What might you be anticipating?

Buttocks: Dreaming about buttocks can indicate primal urges, but also the possibility of being insecure with yourself, whether in body or mind.

Chest: You might feel the need to be protective, possibly of your feelings or opinions. It can also indicate a need for more financial security.

Ears: You should consider listening to others more closely, to hear other points of view, even if they contradict your own. Other opinions are valid.

Ears (falling or cut off): If you lose an ear (or both ears) in a dream, you might be tired of listening to others about something. This might be good or bad, depending on the situation.

Earwax: A dream of cleaning earwax out of your ear can mean that you are resisting others around you, and should open up, "be all ears."

Eyelashes (falling out): Losing your eyelashes often indicates fears about yourself, perhaps a lack of confidence, losing something of importance, or even feeling powerless.

Eyes: Eyes represent knowledge, the intellect, and understanding on the part of the dreamer, and how you use these things in your waking life.

Eyes (bleeding): You might have had to give up a lot for something, or you might be feeling conflicted or pained about a serious issue in your life.

Eyes (closed): If your eyes are closed in a dream, you may be reluctant to see something that you need to see about a person or situation.

Eyes (falling out): If one or both eyes fall out, you might be blinding yourself to something that you should be paying attention to, either in yourself or another.

Eye socket (empty): This ghoulish dream can mean that you refuse to recognize something about yourself, perhaps a negative trait or behavior. Be open to self-reflection and even criticism.

Injury to eye(s): You might be refusing to see what is right in front of you, or you might be feeling hurt in some other way in your waking life.

One eye: You could be unwilling to see another person's point of view, or you might not be looking at a situation in your life clearly.

Feet: Feet can be a symbol of stability, since they literally hold us up! Standing on your feet in a dream speaks to the need to feel rooted and make good choices. Feet can also speak to your need to move, to be free, to travel. You might long to feel more independent, to let your feet carry you away.

Feet (dirty): Feet that are dirty or muddy can indicate that you are feeling stuck in some aspect of your life, unable to move on.

Feet (others'): A dream about another person's feet can indicate that you are too focused on others, what they are doing, and where they are going.

Fingers: Fingers often symbolize ability, both physical and mental, and the confidence to perform needed tasks. They suggest taking action and initiating communication.

Fingers (injured): Cut, broken, or missing fingers can indicate that you are worried about being able to do something in your waking life, feeling that you're not up to the task.

Fingers (pointing): If someone is pointing a finger at you, you might be feeling guilty about something, or fearing that a secret will soon be revealed.

Fingernails (cutting): If you dream about cutting your fingernails, it can mean that you are trying to remove some aspect of yourself, perhaps with the intent of starting something new.

Fingernails (breaking or tearing): A broken or torn fingernail can be a sign of having to deal with situations or people that are annoying, and maybe avoiding them.

Genitals: Genital dreams usually point to your attitudes about your own sexuality, positive or negative. See also "Penis" and "Vagina."

Hand (left): Dreaming of the left hand can indicate being passive (possibly too much), or keeping things hidden, unless you are left-handed. Then see the right hand, below, which applies to you.

Hand (right): A right-hand dream can suggest taking action (or the need to), and doing the right thing. If you are left-handed, see the left hand, above.

Hands (dirty): Dirt or even feces on the hands often points to you feeling "unclean," and wanting to rid yourself of something in your life.

Hands (washing): Washing your hands usually indicates the desire to be cleansed of something, or to take action and leave it behind.

Leg: Legs can symbolize confidence, forward movement, and progress. As with the feet, the legs are responsible for taking you to new places and new situations.

Leg (amputated): Dreaming of an amputated leg suggests that you are trying to cope with the loss of something, which makes you feel weaker and less stable.

Leg (broken): A dream about a broken leg implies that you are experiencing delays and challenges in your life, ones that will require time to overcome.

Legs (crossed): If you are crossing your legs, you might be too defensive in your waking life, too resistant to new ideas and suggestions.

Legs (weak): If your legs feel weak and unable to properly support you, you might be feeling inadequate or lacking in confidence in your waking life.

Lips: Lips often indicate sexual and romantic feelings, especially if they seem inviting. They might be paired in the dream with the mouth (see below).

Mouth: You might need to speak up and express yourself in a clearer way, especially if you are concerned about something and have been saying nothing. Alternately, it's possible that you have already said too much, and might want to keep quiet for the time being.

Mouth (dry): You might not know what to say about a situation in your life. Dry mouth dreams can also indicate that you are simply thirsty in your sleep.

Mouth (covered): If your mouth is covered, you could feel that you are not able to express something important, and thus feel helpless about it.

Mouth (forced shut): If you are unable to open your mouth, you might be trying to keep a secret, or you might feel helpless in some situation, unable to cry out.

Nose: Your nose dream can symbolize a desire to succeed in a chosen task or goal, and/or your need to learn more about a situation in your waking life.

Nose (bleeding): A bloody nose could indicate that you feel attacked or embarrassed in waking life, or that your energy is draining away from stress and other causes.

Nose (blowing): To blow your nose in a dream suggests that you are clearing blockages. You are saying what you need to say, getting it all out.

Nose (falling off): If, weirdly, you see you nose fall off, you might not trust in yourself enough. You will need to in order to move forward.

Penis: The penis relates to sexual drive, energy, fertility, and "manliness," especially if erect, while a flaccid penis might indicate a loss of these things.

Penis (falling off): This dream might indicate a fear of losing your strength, or even your identity, or recognizing those qualities in another instead.

Penis (seeing another's): You might be feeling awkward over approaching someone about a sensitive subject, or it could relate to desires and fantasies.

Toes: Toes can symbolize how you choose to move through your life, with ease or with difficulty, and how much attention you pay to your path.

Toes (losing): If you lose one or more toes, you might be losing your will to continue with something in your life, whether a project, a conviction, or something similar.

Toes (stubbing): Stubbing your toe can mean that you are unsure about continuing with a plan or a decision you've made, but be careful not to self-sabotage.

Toenails (falling off): You might be missing something crucial in a situation you are dealing with, a small but consequential detail.

Toenails (trimming): You could be rethinking something in their life (a decision, a relationship, etc.), or you might need to. Is it time to "trim" something away?

Vagina: A woman dreaming about her own vagina might be thinking more about her sexuality, and how she relates to it, for good or bad.

Vagina (seeing another's): Seeing another vagina can represent the birth of new ideas and plans. If a woman identifies as queer in some way, it might be an expression of her desires and fantasies. A heterosexual man dreaming about a vagina may be in sexual fantasy mode, and the dream might be offering insights into his deeper desires.

BOREDOM

Being bored in your dream can indicate your passion and enthusiasm for something is dwindling, and that it might be time to change things up to get moving again.

BREAK-UPS

As uncomfortable as they are, dreams about break-ups with our partners do happen. Here's what they might indicate:

Break-up (1): You might need to let go of something you've been holding onto (but not necessarily your partner), even if you don't want to.

Break-up (2): Your relationship might be moving into a new stage (not necessarily a break-up) and you will have to help each other in this time of change.

Not breaking up: If you dream that you and your partner have not broken up (when you have in waking life), you are likely in denial about it having happened, and need to face it.

BRIDGE

Bridges obviously connect two points, and dreams about them often center around ideas of connection and movement, as seen in these examples:

Bridge over water: Water indicates emotions, so pay attention to what this dream might be telling you. Are you treading over emotional issues with anxiety or concern?

Crossing a bridge (1): You are at an important point in your life, and need to make a decision about where you will go next, forward or backward?

Crossing a bridge (2): You might be trying to "bridge" the gap between you and someone else, and are willing to take the first steps in doing so.

Crossing a bridge (3): You might be undergoing a major transition in your own life, leaving something old behind and moving onto something new.

Damaged bridge: You could be struggling to connect two parts of your life in a meaningful way, or perhaps you are estranged from someone and need to repair that.

Falling bridge: You might have let something impor-tant get away, or you fear that your life is crumbling, or that you've damaged relations with others.

Falling from a bridge: This dream can represent a fear of failure or indicate a "deep dive" into feelings that you might not want to face, ones that hold you back.

BUCKET

A full bucket can indicate that you are enjoying a full and satisfied life, while an empty bucket suggests that you will triumph over an adversity.

C

CAR

Cars can appear in dreams in a number of ways, with many different possible meanings:

Buying a car: Buying a car in a dream suggests that you feel ready to take on a new responsibility or commitment, possibly a big one.

Car chase: If you are being chased by a car, you might be ignoring something in your life that needs attention. If by police, you might fear someone's authority.

Car crash: A car crash often means that you are experiencing an unexpected setback in your life, one that is frustrating or even infuriating.

Car on fire: A burning car suggests that you are very angry about something in your waking life, and need to address it, to "put out the flames."

Car won't start: If your car won't start no matter what you do, you probably feel frustrated or without power, caused by something in your waking life.

Damaged car: You might well need to be more aware of your surroundings. Someone might be trying to hinder you, or even harm you.

Driving (1): This dream represents your life path and goals and how in control you are. A smooth drive means that you feel in control of your life.

Driving (2): If the road in front of you is rough and difficult, you might not feel fully in control of your life, or you might be facing many difficulties.

Driving off a cliff: A potentially terrifying dream that might be communicating that you feel totally out of control in your waking life and need to take it back.

Driving while lost: You could be feeling adrift and uncertain about your path in life, and still searching for what you want in a career, relationship, or other goal.

Failing brakes: If your brakes fail, you might need to slow down in some area of your life. Perhaps you are moving too fast without considering the consequences.

Hit (or almost hit) by a car: This unsettling dream often suggests an unpleasant experience in your waking life, possibly a conflict with someone that was unexpected.

Hitting someone else: Hitting someone else with a car might indicate that you have hurt someone's feelings, or harmed them in some other way. Or, you worry that you have.

Lost car keys: You are probably feeling stuck and might not be able to continue with something in your life, at least until more information or help (the keys) are acquired.

Overheating car: If the car is overheating, you could be working too hard, and be in danger of burning out. Slow down and reassess.

New car: Dreaming about a new car, or driving one suggests that you are considering taking a new path in life, or already have. Something has recently changed or will.

Parked car: Seeing a parked car might suggest that you need to focus on other things, that this car (plan, idea, relationship) isn't going anywhere.

Passenger in a car: A dream of being the passenger suggests that you don't really feel in control of your life, especially if you're sitting in the back seat.

Stealing a car: If you are stealing the car, you might be trying to take advantage of someone or take credit for something you didn't do.

Stolen or lost car: A stolen car might indicate that you are facing setbacks, or feel that a part of you is being taken away by a person or situation (perhaps a break-up or job loss).

Towed car: A dream of a towed car indicates that something is hindering you, something unexpected that might have come about because you made a mistake.

CAT

Our feline friends often show up in dreams, and their presence has multiple meanings, often to do with the unconscious:

Attacking cat: If a cat attacks you, it might indicate negative behaviors, self-sabotage, gnoring your instincts, or being out of touch with your feminine side.

Cat and dog together: A dream that includes both animals might represent the need to balance your own internal opposites, or better harmonize masculine and feminine traits.

Cat colors: Different cultures attribute different meanings to animal colors; black cats aren't always bad luck! Investigate some of the meanings within your own culture for more clarity.

Cat walks into a room or house: This dream might be an invitation from the unconscious to get in touch with deeper aspects of yourself, especially feminine attributes.

Distressed or angry cat: This dream can mean that you are ignoring some aspect of yourself, a part that needs to be "rescued." What might you be suppressing?

Kittens: A kitten usually represents something new, perhaps a fresh start in life, love, etc. However, a needy kitten might also point to immature behavior.

Sick cat: This dream might be saying that you need to work on balancing your rational and intuitive sides, that something about them is out of balance.

CAVE

A dream cave can symbolize a place of safety or to hide, or also a deeper dive into your unconscious mind, especially if you walk into it.

CELEBRITIES

Dreams about celebrities can come from being a genuine fan, or happen for other reasons:

Friends with a celebrity (1): You might want a better version of the friend or lover you have, or to actually meet the celebrity in question. Realize that both goals might be unattainable.

Friends with a celebrity (2): You also might be trying to make up for something you feel is lacking in your real life, something that you can only have in their dreams.

Intimacy with a celebrity: Affection, kissing, or sexual activity with a celebrity can indicate wish-fulfillment, but also a desire to succeed, and bring what you want into your life.

You are the celebrity: The dream of being a celebrity can point to your own desires for that kind of life.

CHASED

Dreams about being chased (or even doing the chasing) are very common, and don't always point to being afraid:

Chased (1): Being chased in general can mean that you're trying to avoid something in real life. You feel pressure from an issue or a person, and you'd rather not think about it.

Chased (2): You might also fear something about yourself, and you keep running away from it, symbolically speaking. What about yourself might be the cause?

Chased (3): A dream of being chased can indicate your unwillingness to listen to new ideas, or adopt new ways of thinking, doing, and being.

Chased (4): It's also possible that you want to be chased, by a potential romantic partner or a new job offer. Or, maybe you'd like a little more time and space to yourself.

Chased by bees/wasps/hornets: You might be feeling powerless in some situation, or overwhelmed by the enormity of it all, just like a swarm of stinging insects.

Chased by dogs: You could be worried about someone else's aggressive behavior, whether a partner, friend, or co-worker. By all means, look out for danger signs.

Chased by other insects: Ants, beetles, etc., might represent that you are driving yourself too hard, blaming yourself, and/or need to reassess your responsibilities.

Chased by monsters: This dream might point to an old childhood fear, or perhaps your fear of being overwhelmed. Maybe you are also suppressing old feelings and emotions.

Chased by a murderer: You might be dealing with a past or current trauma, or fear that someone or something is trying to take away something from you.

Chased by the police: It's possible that you are feeling guilty about something, or that you are in conflict with an authority figure in your life: a parent, a boss, etc.

Chased by zombies: Is something slowly or subtly threatening you in your waking life? You also might feel trapped or oppressed in some situation or relationship.

Doing the chasing (1): This dream might symbolize your desires and goals, and how much effort you are willing to make to achieve them.

Doing the chasing (2): Alternately, if you are chasing something, you might be frustrated and feel like you're never going to attain it, or that you're falling behind.

CHEATING IN A GAME

Cheating in a game or sport, can mean that you are wrestling with feelings of inadequacy. You might not feel that you are good enough, or you might be lying to yourself.

CHEATING IN A RELATIONSHIP

This unpleasant dream about infidelity can have a variety of explanations:

Cheating (1): You might be feeling guilty about something, or perhaps you feel you have sacrificed your beliefs or your integrity for poor reasons.

Cheating (2): You could desire to expand your horizons and explore your sexuality in new ways, whether within your relationship or not.

Cheating (3): You might be suffering from fears or anxieties about an upcoming major event, such as a marriage, but this dream doesn't mean you will actually be unfaithful.

Partner cheating: You probably fear being abandoned or betrayed, or perhaps you feel that your partner is not giving you enough attention. You might also fear or believe that your partner is not as committed to the relationship as you are.

CHILDHOOD

Dreams about our childhoods can be very complex and have multiple meanings, even if they often speak to our thoughts about our pasts and how they relate to now:

Anxiety: There is something from your past that you have not resolved, and your unconscious mind is reminding you of it, even if you don't wish to hear the message.

Bedroom: You might wish you could have (or return to) a greater sense of safety, and, if happy, this comforting dream might be a way of coping with issues in your adult life.

Childhood crush: You might be longing to complete something you never could, to tell to someone something you never said, or you might feel ready for a new relationship.

Friends: Perhaps you need to reconnect with old friends, or maybe you need to be more aware of old friendship patterns in your current relationships to improve relations.

Neighborhood: If you are feeling a loss of control in your adult life, you might be longing to return to a place that felt safer and more secure, a return to stability and certainty.

Playing: You might wish you could return to a time of innocence, when you had few responsibilities, and could run around and play all day. The good old days!

School: You might have old fears and insecurities that you need to address. That time has moved on, and you need to, as well.

Toys: If you dream about an old beloved toy, you might be needing a break from your stresses and workload, and maybe you want to find new ways to enjoy yourself.

Trauma: It's possible that some trauma is unresolved and needs to be addressed, since you might be ignoring or avoiding it. Consider seeking help from a qualified professional to explore this.

CIGAR

You are feeling relaxed about your life, and on top of things. And while it can be a phallic symbol, as Freud said, it doesn't have to be!

CLOTHING

Clothing represents so much in our waking lives that it's no surprise it does the same in our dreams. Wearing various items of clothing points to many different possible meanings:

Boots: Dreaming about boots can indicate that you are making progress on a project, or are working hard to make something happen ("taking steps").

Bra: You might be in need of more support or protection. You might need to take better care of yourself or focus on your acceptance by others.

Buying clothes: Shopping for clothes can indicate that you have some worries about fitting in with others in a situation and might be trying to "re-clothe" yourself to do it.

Changing clothes: This dream might suggest that you are looking for a new role, one that is a better fit, whether personally or professionally. It's time fora change.

Coat: Wearing a coat (long or short) can speak to your sense of feeling vulnerable, but also might suggest that you feel confident, strong, and in control.

Cross-dressing: Depending on your gender and gender identity, this dream might indicate that there are dormant aspects of yourself that you need to explore, acknowledge, and express.

Dirty clothes: Dirty clothing can represent aspects about yourself that you need to change or clean up, whether habits, beliefs, or personality traits.

Dress: Dreaming about a dress might indicate that you are undergoing an important transformation, or that you need to be aware of how you show yourself to others.

Gloves: Wearing gloves might mean that you are feeling vulnerable or uncertain, and should consider taking some extra measures to protect yourself and establish better boundaries.

Hat: If you are wearing a hat, you might need to exert more control or protect yourself, but you might also simply be feeling confident in your life.

Heels: It's possible that you should be more assertive about something and take control. It's okay to stand up for yourself and raise yourself up to the level of others.

Inappropriate clothing: If what you are wearing is not suitable for the situation, you could be feeling unprepared for something in your waking life.

Inside-out clothing: If your clothes are inside out, you might be a bit of a rebel! You don't like going along with everyone else, and want to form your own opinions.

Jeans: You are probably relaxed and casual about your life right now, happily independent, and/or not afraid of working hard to succeed.

Loose clothing: If your clothes are too loose, you might be suffering from low self-esteem. Maybe you don't feel up to the task, and want to hide from it.

New clothes: Your new clothing might suggest that you are trying to become a new person, or adapt to a new situation. Changes are happening and you might or might not be ready.

Scarf: Wearing a scarf in a dream suggests that you might be trying to protect yourself, or hide your feelings, or even hold back from saying something.

Shoes: Shoes are obviously associated with journeys. Good-fitting shoes indicate that you're comfortable with how your "next step" will proceed. Shoes that don't fit properly suggest that you are feeling held back from making progress, and changes need to be made before you can move on.

Skirt (long): Dreams of skirts of any kind can represent femininity and the desire to embrace those traits, as well as to control them and enjoy your confidence.

Skirt (short): A shorter skirt can mean confidence and willingness to be bold, but also a sense of greater vulnerability and exposure, depending on your comfort level.

Socks: Socks can indicate a longing for comfort and coziness, but also might be pointing out that you're keeping certain thoughts and feelings hidden, perhaps out of fear.

Suit: Your suit dream might be showing that you feel confident and powerful, ambitious and eager for success, but you might fear not being able to live up to others' expectations.

Sunglasses: You might be trying to shield yourself from something unpleasant, or you might be insecure and unwilling to share certain parts of yourself with others.

Swimsuit: If unpleasant, you might be feeling exposed, or dealing with body image concerns. But if nice, you might be reveling in newfound freedoms.

T-shirt: Wearing a t-shirt in a dream could be giving you clues as to how you feel about yourself, and whether or not that self can be accepted by others.

Tie: A tie might indicate that you want to look professional and confident. Psychoanalysts also suggest that a tie is an arrow pointing to one's crotch, so keep that in mind!

Tight clothing: If your clothing is too tight, you are feeling held back and constricted in your waking life, perhaps at work or maybe in a relationship.

Torn clothing: If your clothes are ripped, you might need to rethink your position on a situation. Maybe you need a new angle or rationale.

Trying on clothes (1): If you are trying on formal clothes, you might be preparing for something important, while casual clothes could suggest that you need more relaxation.

Trying on clothes (2): If the clothes fit well, you are probably confident, but if they don't, you might need a boost of confidence in some area of your life.

Wearing black clothing: This dream can indicate issues with your shadow side and unconscious mind, or perhaps your need to fit in with others around you.

Wearing clothing different from everyone else: You might feel like you don't fit in, or that others see you as an outsider.

Wearing the wrong clothes: You probably feel out of place, perhaps even disoriented. Maybe you fear criticism from others or standing out in the crowd too much.

Wearing white clothing: You might have been through difficult times recently and need to put them behind you and move on, to "lighten up."

CLOUDS

Clouds are frequent visitors to many dreams and have different interpretations:

Dark clouds (1): Dark clouds can indicate anger or even depression. You might be facing dark times or sadness and be struggling to cope.

Dark clouds (2): Dark clouds in dreams can also indicate confusion about a situation in your waking life. The answers are "clouded" for now.

White clouds: White clouds suggest brighter times ahead, clarification of difficult or obscure issues, and changes moving into a better time.

COFFEE

The beloved drink can appear in dreams in many ways, and each will suggest different interpretations:

Coffee: Coffee on its own can point to your need to learn more about a person or situation, or perhapsbe a sign that you are moving too rapidly with some issue.

Coffee beans: If you see whole beans in a dream, it might be indicating that you have the potential to succeed at something, and that you have the drive and energy to do it.

Coffee grounds: Coffee grounds sometime indicate that you are wanting a change in your life, or that you must decide about something and don't want to do it.

Drinking coffee with others: If you are drinking coffee with someone, you might be interested in them romantically, or at least, you desire to be more social.

Making coffee: Dreaming about making coffee can suggest obstacles and difficulties in your path, especially if you can't do it. But be careful about being too accommodating.

COLD

Being cold in dreams is as common as feeling warm, and has different interpretations:

Being cold (1): You might be feeling alone or confined in some way, or also "frozen" in place and unable to act, whether in business or in personal matters.

Being cold (2): Are you experiencing emotional distance from someone? Do you need to thaw your relations with them? You dream coldness might be a sign to take action.

Touching something cold: This dream might be a warning that you need to be careful. What is the object and how does it relate to your life?

COLORS

There are countless colors, of course, but here are some of the most common ones and their possible meanings:

Black (1): Black can represent the unknown, the unconscious, the mysterious, an invitation into the darker depths of your psyche, especially if the dream feels positive.

Black (2): In a more negative dream, black can represent fear, hatred, loss of love, death, and sadness. You might be coping with any of these, or are about to.

Black and white: If you dream of these colors together, you might be too rigid in your thinking or approach, seeing things in "black and white." You need to be more flexible.

Blue: Dreams of blue can indicate optimism for the future, as well as feelings of clear thinking, being open, and peace of mind. Sometimes, sadness (feeling "blue") is another meaning.

Brown: Brown is the color of the earth and soil, so a dream of this color might mean that you need to become more grounded, or "go back to your roots."

Gold: A "spiritual" color, gold in a dream can signify rewards (worldly or otherwise), and feeling rich in your life, however that might manifest.

Green (1): The color of growth, rebirth, new life, spring, and much more, this color might be telling you that you need to go ahead with your plans and goals.

Green (2): You might be concerned with the environment, or some aspect of your own personal environment, whether it's related to the earth or not.

Green (3): If the shade of green is a bit darker it might indicate jealousy ("the green-eyed monster"), deception, even cheating on your part or by someone in your life.

Grey: A dream of grey might be warning you about poor health, depression, wasting away, emotional shut-down, or a lack of care and concern.

Orange: Orange in a dream is usually a positive color, indicating friendships, hope, socializing, and your potential gregarious nature.

Pink (1): Pink can symbolize love, affection, a desire for sweet things, and the contentment that love brings. But it can also indicate some immaturity in matters of love.

Pink (2): If the pink feels negative in the dream, you might have unresolved issues with your parents, possibly of codependency or some other unresolved problem.

Purple: Purple can indicate high rank, justice and wealth, as well as devotion and loyalty. You'll need to interpret it according to what else is happening in the dream.

Red (1): Red is energetic, and can indicate drive, energy, passion for something, and sexual urges. How are these things being realized in your waking life?

Red (2): Red can also have negative meanings, such as anger, rage, violence, blood, negative sexual desires. Again, how are these feelings manifesting in your waking life?

Silver: Silver is a color of purification and clarity. It can signify that you crave justice or protection, or that something is protecting you.

Turquoise: A color of healing and emotions, turquoise can mean that you need healing (or are receiving healing of some kind), as well as deeper emotional connection.

White: White is generally a color representing new beginnings, peace, and clarity. Importantly, however, in Asian cultures, white is a color of mourning and death.

Yellow (1): A positive dream of something yellow suggests good use of the mind, making wise choices, being content, and clarity.

Yellow (2): Yellow in a negative dream or context can indicate feelings of betrayal, illness, cowardice, and deception, whether on your part or on the part of someone in your life.

COMBING YOUR HAIR

You could need more organization and order in your life and mind, or you might be trying to find out important information about some situation.

COMPUTERS

Computers dominate our waking lives, so it's not surprising that they will show up in our dreams in various ways:

Buying a computer: You might be expecting a promotion at work, a raise, or some other advancement. If you aren't expecting these, keep your eyes open, anyway!

Computer (1): Of course, computers represent our interactions with technology in the modern world, and our need to keep up with the ever-changing tech landscape.

Computer (2): Alternately, a computer might symbolize that you are becoming too robotic, or are letting others make your choices for you. Reclaim your individuality and feelings!

Computer game: If you're playing a game, you might be too focused on yourself and your own life. Perhaps it's time to turn your attention outward a little more.

Computer keyboard: You are trying to communicate with someone or with a group of people. There is some-thing important that you need to say, an idea whose time has come.

Computer keyboard (broken): You might be afraid that something is about to go from bad to worse, or that legal problems are involved with the situation.

Computer virus: Has something in your life recently "crashed"? You might also be ignoring friends and family, potentially even damaging those relationships.

Frozen computer: You might be worried that something is going to delay or ruin your plans. This could be because of interference from a boss, or someone else in your life.

Laptop: You have a need to connect with others for some reason. This might be because of an idea, the need to be more social, or because you have to make a decision.

Stolen computer/laptop: You might be relying too much on your computer, or your "virtual" life, or relying on others' help, instead of doing things for yourself.

CONFUSION

If you are feeling confused or surrounded by confusing images, you might be facing different options in real life and don't know which one to choose.

COOKING

To dream about cooking suggests that you might be wanting to influence others to like/love you, or perhaps you want to express your feelings of care to others.

CRIME

Crime shows up in different ways in dreams, and you might be either the victim or the perpetrator, though being the victim is more common:

Being mugged: You might be dealing with having to do something that is not in your nature, or you are struggling to find your true identity in a given situation.

Being scammed/conned: You are probably worried that someone is taking advantage of you in your waking life. You could mistrust that person until you know better.

Breaking into a house: If you are breaking into a house, you might need more answers to a perplexing situation, or you are trying to learn more about yourself. Or both.

Car break-in: If someone is breaking into your car, you might be frustrated about how something is going. Your plans have been derailed, or "highjacked."

House break-in (1): Something from your unconscious might be revealing itself; perhaps you have been denying it, but it will no longer be ignored.

House break-in (2): You might fear that your personal space is being invaded too much, or that you are losing your sense of self because of another.

Kidnapped: You are probably feeling trapped in some situation, and unsure of how to get out of it.

Kidnapping: If you are the kidnapper, you could be holding onto something (a person, an idea, the past) too hard. Also, try not to force your ideas onto others.

Murder victim: If you are being murdered, something important has probably come to an end in your life, and you are struggling to cut ties with it, or just to accept the fact.

Murdering someone: If you are the murderer, you might desire to put an old habit or belief behind you. It's possible that you are suppressing your anger about it.

Taken hostage: You could be struggling with feelings of powerlessness and having no options in some situation or relationship in your waking life.

Terrorism victim: You might be fearing the anger of someone in your life, or of having to confront them about something, and seeing their unhappy reaction.

Terrorist: If you are committing a terrorist act, you could be struggling with your own anger and frustration about something, and feeling the need lash out.

Victim of some other theft: A person or project might be wasting your time, and you are feeling robbed of that time. Or, someone might be taking credit for your ideas and work.

Witnessing a crime: To see a crime being committed in your dream can mean that you feel powerless to do something about a situation in your life.

D

DANCING

Dancing is a fun activity that many people enjoy. Here's what it might mean if you do it in a dream:

Asking someone to dance: You are probably more of a take-charge person, who leads and charts the course, or maybe you want to be and are working on that.

Attending a dance: You have or want to have happiness and joyful times in your life. This dream can speak to your need for pleasure and a sense of belonging.

Being asked to dance: This dream could indicate that you tend to follow, rather than lead, or that you are searching for directions and help.

Child dancing: This dream can suggest that your inner child is happy and doing well. It can also reflect your satisfaction with your family, if you have children.

Dancing (1): You are probably feeling freer about your life now, less inhibited and more able to simply enjoy yourself. Enjoy the feeling!

Dancing (2): Dancing can represent the physical body, including sexual wants and needs. How do you relate to your body at this point? What more do you want or need?

Dancing with a partner: If you know the person, it probably represents your closeness to them, whether a partner or a friend. If you don't know the person, this dream might represent that you are more at peace with yourself and your inner dualities.

Dancing with an ex: Oddly, this dream often means that you have come to terms with the breakup, and are happy for that person. You can now enjoy the next chapter.

Dancing with the dead: Not an indicator of death, but rather a possible reflection of your memories of someone in your past and how they still make you feel.

DAYS OF THE WEEK

The days of the week show up in dreams fairly commonly, and each day has different meanings. These might be enhanced if the dream about a given day happens on that particular day:

Sunday: Sunday in a dream might indicate that you want to relax (or need more relaxation), and perhaps you are actively looking for ways to do it.

Monday: A Monday often signifies a new beginning, and can be telling you that now is the time to take action and start something or deal with a problem.

Tuesday: Dreaming about Tuesday might be telling you to make plans and give them their full attention. Your goal can be attained with work.

Wednesday: A Wednesday dream might be a reflection that you are feeling conflicted, stressed, even miserable about something. But keep going and a solution will be found.

Thursday: A dream about Thursday suggests that there is something in your life that needs your attention, or that you need to pay closer attention to something than you are.

Friday: You might be coming to the end of a project or situation, and you can feel confident that it is complete and that all well be well.

Saturday: A Saturday can represent new opportunities or a sign that the decisions that you are making now will turn out in your favor.

DEAD

Seeing the dead in dreams is probably as old as humanity. Many view it as a sign from their departed, but these dreams can have many meanings:

Ancestor: If you see someone long dead, such as an ancestor, it might be pointing to something in your life that needs to "die" and be let go of.

Dead are alive again: Often, seeing someone dead who is alive again in your dream can mean that you have unfinished business with them, perhaps things left unsaid or undone.

Dead asking for clothing: Do you need to cover for someone? Protect them? Or did you need to do this for someone who has passed?

Dead asking for food: You might feel obligated to "feed" the person in question, with answers, love, revelations, things you might not have thought about before.

Dead asking for money: You might need to offer more to the others in your life, whether that is kindness, protection, financial aid, love, or encouragement.

Dead asking for water: There could be something unfinished between the two of you, especially as it relates to emotions. You also might need to "drink" from the well of your unconscious.

Dead body in a coffin: It can seem morbid, but this dream suggests that you will soon "bury" a problem that you have been trying to solve and put it away for good.

Dead body in your home: There might be something negative about you that you are not aware of, something that is "dead weight" and holding you down.

Dead children: If you see a child of yours who has passed, you are likely unable to accept that death. This is normal, but you should seek counseling from a qualified professional.

Dead parents: If a dead parent appears in your dream, you might have left some things unsaid, or are still holding onto them to deal with that loss.

Dead person who says nothing: You could have emotional or spiritual blocks to something, or perhaps you need to pay more attention to non-verbal communication in your life.

Dead relatives and friends: You might be hoping to go back and enjoy an experience with someone who has passed on, especially if you were close in life.

Gift of clothing: If someone dead give you clothing, you could be seeking protection, warmth, and some assurances for the uncertainties in your life.

Gift of food: You might desire more energy and some kind of "nourishment for the soul" to help you through a difficult time.

Gift of money: This dream can be a message that you have all of the gifts you need already, and that these riches are love, wisdom, belonging, and knowledge.

Gift of water: Water is often connected to emotional states in a dream, so this dream might be telling you to dive into the ocean of your unconscious to cleanse yourself.

Phone calls: If someone dead phones you, pay attention to what they say to you and how you respond. It might be your unconscious mind trying to tell you something important.

Speaking with the dead (1): Talking with someone who is dead (that you don't know) can be a sign that you are being influenced by others, and not for the better.

Speaking with the dead (2): You might be dealing with a loss of some kind (a death, a relationship, a job), and are trying to find ways to cope with it.

Wanting you to follow: If a dead person wants you to go with them, you might not understand why they died, or you might be feeling very alone and looking for comfort.

DEAD END

Something is not working, or is blocking you, and you need to find a new way forward. Or, a job, a relationship, or a friendship might be coming to an end.

DEATH

Death is an enormous topic with many different aspects, evoking all kinds of feelings. Deaths in dreams have numerous meanings, from actual death to big changes and transitions:

Buried alive: You might well be resisting change, or feeling stuck in some situation that you cannot get out of.

Dead body: To dream of a dead body might be telling you that there is "dead weight" in your life that needs to be disposed of.

Death in a car crash: You might be feeling that your ambition or "drive" is dying, or at least coming to a halt, perhaps unexpectedly.

Death in a plane crash: A common death dream that often speaks to your fear of failure, and that your goals are failing to work out, that they won't get anywhere.

Death of a child: This upsetting dream (especially if of one of your own children) might actually be pointing to the need for you to let go of something in your past.

Death of a friend or loved one: You might be lacking something in yourself that you see in that other person, and you perceive it as something you need.

Death of a parent: You might be reaching a point in your life where your relationship with one or both of your parents needs to change to be better for everyone.

Death of a pet: You could be facing the painful end of something you don't want to lose, such as a job, a relationship, a home, etc.

Death of a spouse: You might be worried that your spouse will leave you, or that unsaid things still need to be spoken while both of you are still here.

Death of a stranger: If you dream of seeing an unknown person die, you might be feeling detached from a friend or life, and need to work to renew ties.

Drowning: You could be feeling overwhelmed by your emotions and feelings, and fear drowning in them, or being unable to control them.

Dying in a dream (1): Dying in a dream in general can mean that you are undergoing a major shift or transition into something new, and that change is on the way.

Dying in a dream (2): More negatively, you might be feeling trapped and upset by someone or a situation and you are looking for a way out of it.

Dying in a dream (3): You might fear actual death, or the unknown. You could have an impending sense of doom, whether this is the case in waking life or not.

Dying in childbirth: A pregnant woman might have this dream in genuine fear for her safety, but for anyone, it can mean the old is dying off so that the new can be born.

Faking one's death: If you pretend to die in a dream, you might be looking for a big change in your waking life, a chance to reinvent yourself.

Nearly dying: To dream about narrowly escaping death suggests that you might be falling back into old habits and ways of living, but also that you have the chance to start again.

DICE

If you are rolling dice in a dream, you might be taking unnecessary chances in your life, maybe even tempting fate. Be careful not to gamble too much.

DISEASE

Having a disease can be a disturbing dream that can point to waking-life health issues or fears, but also has other meanings:

Disease (1): If you are dealing with a real-life disease, this dream might simply reflect that, as well as your anxieties around it.

Disease (2): You might be struggling with anxiety and emotional issues in general, but be careful that you don't let these consume you; despair is not the best solution!

Infection: What emotions and thoughts are you internalizing? Are they eating away at you? What can you do to "purge" them in a healthy way?

Terminal disease (1): You might be afraid of your own mortality, and feel that you need to start living more, savoring every moment.

Terminal disease (2): You could be wrestling with feelings of hopelessness and/or self-pity, as if there is nothing more you can do, but remember, there always is.

DISGUST

If something disgusts you in a dream, you might be dealing with an unhealthy situation, and you need to work to get out of it. You might also be ashamed of something.

DOCUMENTS

Reading or viewing documents in your dream can suggest that you might be privy to important information, or that you are going to have an insight.

DOG

Dogs are a common animal found frolicking in our dreams, and can carry many meanings:

Attacking dog: A dog bite might indicate a sense of betrayal from someone close, while being chased by a dog often means that you are running away from something.

Black dog: In folklore, black dogs were seen as warnings or signs of evil, but for your dream, it might mean that you need to connect more with your shadow side.

Friendly dog: Dogs are often seen as signs of protection for dreamers, so this might indicate that you feel watched over and taken care of.

Puppies: A puppy can suggest optimism for the future and for your personal growth, but also that you might have underdeveloped masculine qualities.

Sick or injured dog: An injured dog might represent you and convey the need to heal, or to uncover masculine wounds or psychological issues.

DOOR

Doors often feature in dreams and are filled with symbolic meanings. Here are some of the most common ones:

Broken door or door knob: You might need something else to get you to the next step in your life, but it is missing at the moment, or it doesn't work.

Closed door: A closed door can represent an obstacle, though not necessarily a permanent one. It can also symbolize the ending of something.

Door knob: A door knob can represent a key element or tool that you need to make something happen, and it is probably already available to you.

Door opening away from you: You are ready to delve within and do some inner work with yourself, and maybe learn more about yourself in the process.

Door opening toward you: You probably want to be open to people and more accepting and welcoming, perhaps more hospitable.

Doorbell: A doorbell can suggest that you want to enjoy new experiences, or perhaps that you are already being presented with them and need a reminder.

Doormat: You might feel as if people are taking advantage of you, or "walking all over you." Does the doormat say anything? How is this significant for you?

Entering a doorway: If you enter through a doorway, you are probably feeling prepared to take the next step in some aspect of your life, whether personal or professional.

Front door: Seeing a front door (yours or another's) might indicate that you want to keep out the world for now, and maybe keep away certain people from your personal space.

Locked door: Someone or something might be blocking you at the moment, preventing you from moving forward. Or, you might be unable to take advantage of certain opportunities.

Locked in: If you are locked inside, there is something about yourself that you need to examine and learn from. You're not allowing yourself some freedoms.

Locked out: If you are locked out, you might be feeling the need to stay away from people for a while. You are more important that whatever's happening inside.

Locking a door: If you are locking a door, you might be shutting yourself away from others, and denying yourself chances to make friends, move ahead, and so on.

Locking a door (unable): If you want to lock a door but can't, you might be feeling that others are in your space too much and you need to retreat.

Open door: You are probably open to new ideas and opportunities, and ready to engage in new ways of doing things, whether personally or professionally.

Opening and closing a door: This dream can symbolize that you have opportunities, but you will have to wait for the right moment to take them, to walk through.

Revolving doors. You might feel as if you are chasing your tail and not making progress. Or perhaps things in your life come and go and never seem permanent.

Several doors: You likely have many choices before you, and will need to decide which is the best. Are some doors open and some closed? That could provide clues.

Slamming a door shut: If someone slams a door on you, you might be feeling ignored or denied. Maybe you want to be a part of something, but can't at this time.

Standing in a doorway (1): If someone else is standing in a doorway, are they a friend or foe? Are they here to help you or to hinder you?

Standing in a doorway (2): If you are standing in a doorway, you might be weighing whether to move ahead with some plan or decision and are hesitating to decide.

Unlocked door: An unlocked door most often implies opportunities, signifying that the way forward is clear, if you choose to step through.

DREAMING

If you happen to dream that you are dreaming, you could be very worried about a certain situation, and are trying to put an extra layer up in your mind for self-protection.

E

ELEVATOR

Dreams about elevators often represent change, personal growth, and periods of transition. Whether the elevator is going up or down may symbolize how you feel about these changes.

EMBARRASSMENT

If you feel embarrassment, you are possibly dealing with a lack of self-confidence in your real life, whether professional or personal, especially sexual insecurity.

ENGAGEMENT

You might dream of getting engaged, but it's not always about marriage:

Breaking off an engagement: If you dream of breaking off an engagement, you might have made a poor decision about something and are now regretting it, or wishing you could change it.

Engagement (1): If you are unmarried, you might be feeling ready to commit to someone, whether to a real person or just to the idea in general.

Engagement (2): You could be feeling lonely and looking for companionship or long-term security in the form of a commitment and promise. What are you missing in your life?

ENVELOPE

An envelope may indicate impending news or communication coming your way. What are you hoping or fearing will be inside?

ESP

Dreaming about having ESP (extrasensory perception) or being psychic might be a message to trust your instincts more. Go with your gut and your feelings on the situation you have in mind.

EXERCISE

Exercising in a dream often means that you have some concerns about your health (and want to improve it), or that you worry about your body image and/or your self-esteem.

EXIT

To dream of an exit or an exit sign might be telling you that you are looking for a way out of some situation in your life.

EXPLOSION

An explosion in a dream is generally indicative of some kind of stress in your waking life. It may also symbolize repressed emotions reaching their breaking point.

F

FABRIC

Fabric can represent your creative side and/or how you "weave" the strands of your own life together. Consider the color of the fabric, as well. See "Colors."

FALLING

Falling from a great height, such as from a building or an airplane, can signify insecurity, lack of confidence, or a loss of control. You might fear unknown circumstances, be facing upcoming challenges, or feel overwhelmed.

FAME

Dreaming about being famous can indicate a desire for more recognition, or a need for acknowledgement. It might also reveal a fear of failure or lack of success.

FAMILY

Family dreams are at the top of the list for many people, and depending on your relationships with them, they have a variety of different interpretations:

Aunt: An aunt in a dream can indicate things you both like and dislike about yourself, and/or the need for mothering of some kind, even if not from your actual mother.

Brother: If you have a good relationship, you probably have a bond. If bad, unresolved issues. If the person is unknown to you, you are possibly seeking brotherly advice and protection.

Brother-in-law: You might be afraid of tensions in the family, with in-laws or others, and perhaps a feeling of disconnect with people who are "new" family.

Cousin: You might be looking for stronger ties with those who are not close relatives, or fearing that such a connection is not there.

Daughter: You could be feeling a sense of protection toward her or someone else, or perhaps you are the one who needs to feel protected and nurtured, by yourself and others.

Daughter-in-law: This dream can mean that something has happened or will happen that is unexpected and might cause you happiness or distress, depending on the situation.

Father: Depending on your relationship with him, this dream can reflect your sense of security, and possibly your own ability to step up and take charge of a situation.

Father-in-law: You might be questioning your own authority, and your ability to make decisions, or your relationship with another authority figure in your life (such as a boss).

Granddaughter: You could be in a reflective state about the passage of time, and wondering if you have done enough for your granddaughter (if you have one) or others.

Grandfather: You might be thinking about your own stability and longevity, as well as what you can learn from the past (your own and the past in general).

Grandmother: How do you view your own background and your own family's history? Can you take comfort in what has come before? What advice and guidance do you need?

Grandson: You might be thinking about your own legacy, what you will leave behind for others, and/or perhaps fearing that you will not measure up to expectations.

Mother: This dream will reflect your own relationship with your mother, good or bad, and how you feel nurtured and taken care of, or how you care for yourself.

Mother-in-law: This dream is asking what relationship you have to this person, or even your mother. It might also indicate that we need to continue with our efforts, whatever they might be.

Nephew: You could be asking how important your relationship with your family is, and if you can strengthen ties with relatives, both close and more distant.

Niece: You might need more connection (with a real-life niece or others), but also more happiness and relaxation in your life. Be more appreciative of others.

Sister: This dream can be a reflection of a strong tie you have to someone, whether your sister or someone else. Or, it might be someone who is no longer in your life that you miss.

Sister-in-law: This dream might give you clues about how you view your partner's family, and whether you need to strengthen or loosen those ties. Or it might indicate someone you admire.

Son: Depending on whether the dream seems positive or negative, it can shed light on your own emotional needs, your confidence or your insecurities.

Son-in-law: Dreaming about a son-in-law can indicate that you are comfortable just going along with the situation and not causing dissent or problems.

Uncle: A dream about an uncle can represent your need to remain true to what you believe in, but also perhaps to know when to throw in the towel on something.

FEAR

To be afraid in a dream almost certainly indicates fear of something in waking life. This might suggest anxiety, self-doubt, self-preservation, irrational fears, and other kinds of fear.

FINDING

Dreams of finding and discovering usually occur when you are searching for something in your life:

Finding someone: You might have recently discovered something new about someone in your life. This could be good or bad, depending on the nature of the dream.

Finding something: Something important might be about to change in your life, possibly something you were looking for all along. Also, you could be discovering things about yourself that you never knew, or getting into better contact with your own unconscious mind.

Unable to find something: You might be struggling with your direction or your purpose, or even who you really are. What are you looking for in your dream?

FIRE

Fire will have many different interpretations (good and bad), depending on how it is seen in a dream:

Dreamer is on fire: You might feel attacked by others, that you're being "flamed." Or, you might have done something to incur the anger of someone, even if accidentally.

Escaping from a fire: You might be trying to get away from something dangerous in your life, or you might be ignoring something that can no longer be avoided.

Fire and smoke: Seeing both together in a dream might indicate that things are out of control in your life. Danger might be recent or on the way.

Fire and water: If both elements are present in a dream, it might be that you are facing a conflict, being tugged in opposite directions by two opposing forces.

Fire without fear: Viewing a fire without fear can indicate that you are burning away the old to make way for the new. Transformation is possible.

Forest fire: A forest fire can represent a separation from your unconscious mind, but also anger at damage being done to the earth, and feeling helpless about it.

House fire: You might need to change something about yourself or your life, especially if it's your house.

Putting out a fire: You are beginning to take action to stop a danger or threat in your life, before it gets out of control. You probably already have the means to do so.

Starting a fire: You might have anger that you are trying to suppress, symbolized by the flames that erupt when you make a fire in your dream.

Surrounded by fire: You could be trapped in a situation, or you might be willing to take too many risks to get out of something.

FISHING

If you are fishing, you might be allowing old feelings to resurface in your life. Or you could be trying to "catch" an answer, a decision, or even a compliment.

FLAT TIRE

Dreaming of a flat tire or tires, suggests that you are losing your drive for something, slowing down, unable to continue. See also "Cars."

FLYING

A common and sometimes exhilarating dream, flying can be thrilling or terrifying, depending on the dream:

Fear of falling while flying: If you are afraid, it can mean that you are controlled by fears, have anxiety, or have trouble letting go. You need to examine these fears.

Flying downward: Flying toward the ground might indicate that you want a deeper connection with yourself, or perhaps with your unconscious mind.

Flying low or hovering: Hovering or keeping near to the ground suggests that you are or want to be more grounded, and perhaps that you have a determined attitude.

Flying over buildings and houses: Sometimes occurring in lucid dreams, these images can mean that you have or want more control of yourself or your surroundings.

Flying upward: If you tend to fly upward in your dreams, it suggests expansion, spiritual awakening, or perhaps the broadening of your horizons.

Trying to fly and failing: You might feel held back by something, or lack the confidence needed to move forward, take a risk, or get "unstuck."

FOG

To see fog rolling in while dreaming often means that you are uncertain, confused, and lost. You might not be seeing the whole picture and thus need to proceed with caution.

FOOD

Food is such an important part of our lives that it's no surprise that our favorite (and not-so-favorite) foods often enter our dreams:

Apple: You might be due for a reward of some kind, or you might be thinking about your health and considering getting a checkup from a doctor.

Bacon: Dreaming of bacon might mean that you are enjoying, or perhaps craving, a grounded and stable life, one that is satisfying and nourishing.

Banana: A banana in a dream can mean abundance, fertility, even good luck and new opportunities, but it can also indicate the need to resist temptation.

Banana peel: If you dream about a banana peel, you could be wrestling with insecurities and the fear of "slipping" and losing control of a situation. Take greater care.

Birthday cake: This dream might indicate that you are celebrating something, or making a successful passage or achievement, with the promise of more to come.

Bread: You could be dreaming about your basic needs, and what those mean to you. What comforts and necessities are the most important and how do you keep them?

Breakfast: Something new might be about to start in your life, but be sure to continue to nourish and prepare yourself before you start it. Maybe you're just anticipating your real breakfast!

Butter: Butter in a dream often means contentment in life. Or it might mean that you are still looking for that contentment and might need to change some things to acquire it.

Cake: Cakes can have several meanings, but often speak to the need for you to share more with others, not only the good things, but also workloads and burdens.

Candy: Candy can indicate that you enjoy taking pleasure in the simple things in life, or it might mean you are being tempted by something forbidden.

Cheese: Cheese dreams often symbolize finances, such as income and even windfalls, and the need to have enough money to live and feel secure.

Chocolate: Chocolate in a dream can indicate the need to reward yourself now and then, but it can also mean that you're indulging a bit too much and should ease up.

Coconut: Coconuts symbolize wealth and money, and to dream of one often means you are expecting money and abundance, or at least you hope for it.

Cookies: If you dream about cookies, you might be longing for something pleasant, but you might also be overindulging, or letting trivial troubles bother you too much.

Dessert: A dessert dream suggests that you are enjoying a well-earned reward, and perhaps want to celebrate. Or, perhaps you are giving into temptation too much?

Eggs: Eating eggs can represent new birth, ideas, and potential. Scrambled eggs can mean that you have to deal with the consequences of something you've done.

Fig: Dreaming about figs suggests that something positive is about to happen, or that you want this. Figs have sexual connotations, as well.

Fish: Fish as food in a dream can mean you are having deep thoughts about your spirituality and your knowledge.

Fruit: Dreaming about fruit in general often indicates abundance and financial prosperity, as well as sexual desire. Or perhaps you are thinking about having a child.

Garlic: You are probably a practical person, who will take measures to protect yourself and overcome your difficulties.

Grapes: A bunch of grapes suggest that you are working hard and will be rewarded for your efforts. Grapes often represent abundance and prosperity.

Ham: If you dream about eating ham, your unconscious might be telling you to hold back a bit, conserve energy, and look after your emotions.

Ice cream: Ice cream can be telling you to enjoy the moment, or it might be saying that you need to cool down your anger about something and "chill out."

Jam: Jam of any kind suggests that you are making interesting new discoveries, but it might also mean that you have gotten yourself into a "sticky" situation.

Lemons: A lemon can indicate that you think something is of poor quality, or you might need to "clean out" some things from your life.

Lettuce: If you are eating lettuce in a dream, you might need to look at your diet and see if you are getting enough greens. Or perhaps something else needs nourishment.

Meat: Meat in general indicates that you want to get to the core of something, to understand it, or perhaps you feel that someone else has what you want.

Muffins: If you bake and/or eat a muffin in a dream, you are probably a hard worker who wants to enjoy the fruits of your labor, especially the finer things in life.

Mushrooms: If you eat mushrooms, you might feel powerful, but just seeing them (such as growing from the ground) could indicate that you need to rethink some of your decisions.

Nuts: Nuts can indicate success and acquiring what you desire, or that you think a situation is crazy or confusing (it's "nuts").

Onion: An onion in a dream might mean that you need to "peel away the layers" of a situation to learn more about it. You are seeking answers to some question or problem.

Orange: If you are eating an orange, you are probably happy with where you are in your life right now.

Oysters: If you dream about eating oysters, you might be pursuing pleasures that are perverse and unsavory, or at least beneath you. Think about your morals.

Pie: This dream can mean that you want your fair share, your "piece of the pie." Be careful not to overdo things when striving for it, however.

Potato: The humble potato suggests that you are feeling grounded, even earthy, but be careful about becoming lazy or a "couch potato."

Raisins: Surprisingly, eating raisins in a dream can mean that you feel attacked or negated. Perhaps it is a person, or maybe a situation, that is older and/or inhibiting.

Rice: If you see or eat rice in a dream, it often symbolizes joy, prosperity, happiness, a good domestic life, and even good luck. You have or want these things.

Salt: Dreaming of salt speaks to your sense of self, often that you are feeling confident, or perhaps that you are experiencing a resurgence of self-esteem and enthusiasm.

Sandwich: Eating a sandwich might indicate that you are feeling pressure from two opposing forces, which are "sandwiching you in." Or, you need to deal with two things at the same time.

Steak: Eating a steak in a dream might be a sign that you need to trust yourself more, especially your gut and your instincts.

Strawberries: Strawberries can indicate sexuality, especially feminine sexuality, as well as desire, fantasy and temptation. How are you enjoying them?

Tomatoes: If you are eating a tomato in a dream, it can symbolize that you either have or are looking forward to good health.

Vegetables: Dreaming about vegetables in general symbolizes nourishment of all kinds—physical, spiritual, emotional, etc.—and your need for each of these.

Watermelon: Watermelons are often symbolic of love and lust, and interestingly, pregnant women seem more likely to dream about them.

G

GENDER/SEX SWAPS

To dream about being a different sex/gender indicates that you might be ignoring a part of yourself, perhaps feminine or masculine traits that need to be better integrated.

GENIE

What are you hoping and wishing for? Or what have you done ("the genie out of the bottle") that now cannot be undone?

GHOST

Ghosts can be scary, but in dreams, they are not always the stuff of nightmares. They can symbolize several things:

Becoming a ghost: You are likely trying to escape from some situation in your life, and you wish you could just disappear, or at least not be noticed anymore.

Chased by a ghost (1): If the ghost is not so threatening, something from your past or unconscious is probably reaching out to you, trying to get your attention.

Chased by a ghost (2): If the ghost intends to harm you, it might be telling you that you are ready to face something in your life (especially from your past) and put it to rest.

Ghost: It's possible that a goal or desire of yours is no longer available to you, and the thought of this might "haunt" you until you face up to it. Alternately, it might be time for you to leave something behind you, or put to rest the "ghosts in your past," so that you can truly move on.

Ghost in a basement: Your unconscious might be harboring something, like repressed memories, that nevertheless come up to haunt you on occasion.

Ghost in a bedroom: You could be struggling with intimacy issues, or feeling that you are not completely safe in a relationship. Something disturbs your sense of security.

Ghost in a closet: What are you hiding about yourself. This could be anything from secrets to your sexuality. Is it something you want or need to reveal?

Ghost in a dining room: To see a ghost in a communal living space can indicate that you are dealing with family issues and dynamics.

Ghost in an attic: What have you put away and forgotten about? Are there some things stored in your mind that need to be taken out and re-examined?

Ghost possession: If a ghost tries to possess you, you are probably struggling to feel in control of your life right now, maybe even "invaded" by outside forces.

Ghost of a dead relative or friend: You might be feeling guilt or regret over how you related to this person while they were alive. You wish to say things you didn't.

Ghost of a living relative or friend: You could possibly be afraid of this person right now, worried that they intend you some ill will.

Ghost of yourself: You might worry about your own mortality, or perhaps some aspect of yourself that even scares you.

Trying to touch a ghost: Often your hand simply passes through, which indicates that you are not quite ready to deal with past hurts or traumas, even though you want to. Have patience!

GLASS

Glass of all kinds shows up in dreams often, with several possible meanings:

Breaking glass: If glass breaks or shatters in your dream, you might be experiencing a breakthrough of some kind, even a victory on your part.

Broken glass (car): You might have found that something is causing problems for you in moving ahead with some plan. Your view of how to proceed is now obscured.

Broken glass (on the floor): Glass pieces lying on the floor can sometimes indicate issues with someone who has broken their word. Now you must clean up the mess.

Broken glass (window): It might be that you are feeling vulnerable, that something about your inner life has been exposed or is threatened.

Dirty glass: Perhaps obviously, you are probably having trouble seeing a situation clearly. You need to do some clean-up to get a better view.

Eating or chewing glass (1): You might have said something that was hurtful to someone else. You've cut them with your words and they are offended, angry, or even sad.

Eating or chewing glass (2): Are you struggling to find the right words to say to someone? You might fear coming across in the wrong way.

Glass (1): You could be attempting to stay behind a barrier for your own emotional protection, but still want to be able to see others.

Glass (2): Alternately, you might be exposing more of yourself and you feel comfortable about doing that, about letting people see you from the outside.

Walking on broken glass: You are likely in pain in some way, and have to find out how to navigate through it, one step at a time.

GRAVEYARD

Dreaming about a graveyard can symbolize those parts of the self that you have set aside or ignored. It can also mean that you are mourning something.

GUEST

A dream about a guest will likely have two different meanings:

Receiving a guest: You are open to new situations, people, and activities, unless the guest is unwanted, then you are closing yourself off and need more solitude.

You are the guest: You might be dealing with an issue in your life (good or bad) that will not last. It will eventually move on, whether you want it to or not.

GUN

Since a gun is a weapon, these dreams often have aggressive or even negative connotations, depending on the situation:

Gun (1): A gun in your dream can indicate anger or aggression, and perhaps the need to protect yourself from dangers, real or imagined.

Gun (2): You might feel strong, ready to handle some situation, to take charge and not back down from intimidation.

Gun (3): In the Freudian sense, the gun can represent the penis, and you will have to evaluate how that imagery works in your life and what it might mean.

Gun fails to fire: You might feel powerless about something, unable to tackle it, or you might have sexual doubts and fears.

Shooting a gun: If you shoot someone, it often indicates repressed anger. If the victim exists in real life, you are probably angry or hostile toward that person.

Shot by a gun: If you are the one who is shot, you might feel attacked or victimized in your life, especially if the shooter actually exists. It's time to address the problem.

H

HALLWAY

There might be aspects of yourself you haven't explored enough yet, especially if the hall is empty. Or, it can mean that you are embarking on a new path.

HAPPINESS

Dreaming about being happy might, paradoxically, mean that you are actually not, but want to be. You will need to examine how best to cultivate happiness in your life.

HAUNTED HOUSE

To dream that you buy or live in a haunted house suggests that you might be running away from the past, but the "ghosts" of old feelings and problems will still catch up with you.

HEAT

If you feel heat from any source, you might be embarrassed about something in waking life, or perhaps passionate, angry, or some mixture of all of these feelings.

HEAVINESS

If you struggle to move under your own weight (or under an external weight), you are doing too much, or working too hard. Lighten the load and try to relax.

HOLIDAYS AND SPECIAL OCCASIONS

There are many different holidays all around the world, and each has specific meanings for a dreamer. Here are some of the most common and universal ones:

Birthday (1): To dream about your birthday suggests that you are happy and accepting of yourself, and where you are at this point in your life.

Birthday (2): Alternately, dreaming about your birthday (especially if the dream is not pleasant) might be a reflection of your fear of growing older.

Christmas: Christmas dreams often symbolize family, togetherness, happiness. If you have negative feelings about the season, this dream might indicate your longing for such things.

Easter: This dream can signify that you are moving past a difficult problem or time, and that newer and better things are on the way.

Halloween: You might be trying to hide a part of yourself (wearing a mask or costume), to put on a new face, or you are having difficulty accepting something about yourself.

New Year's Day/Eve: You are about to begin something new, and have optimism about it, or you want to and are working on bringing it about.

HORIZONTAL LINE

A horizontal line in a dream can often mean that your main focus currently is on the worldly and the concrete, rather than the ideal or spiritual.

HORSE

Horses can represent many different things in a dream, most often to do with feelings of freedom and sexuality:

Dark or black horse: A dark-colored horse often symbolizes the mysterious, the wild. It can represent male sexual energy, or the need to take the plunge into the unknown.

Dead horse: Something you have relied upon is now gone. It can no longer help you the way it once did. Don't "beat a dead horse" over it.

Herd of horses: A herd of horses can indicate that you are dealing with uncontrolled feelings or urges, which are "running wild" in your mind.

Horse running toward you: This dream might be communicating that you are waiting for some important information, a letter, a phone call, etc., perhaps impatiently.

Riding a horse: You might feel free and unrestrained, perhaps ready to try something new, take a new job, find a new sexual partner, and so on.

Standing horse (1): To see a horse standing in a dream can indicate strength, power, or sexual potency, whether your own or someone else's.

Standing horse (2): Another interpretation of seeing a horse is that you might be arrogant or foolish, and you might need to take things more seriously.

White horse: White horses can suggest that something good has come into your life, something beneficial, or even beautiful, whether a person, a situation, or something else.

Wild horse(s): A wild horse or horses can represent your desire to be free of some burden or responsibility, especially if you manage to ride the horse.

HOUSE

Houses are very common in dreams and have a multitude of possible meanings:

Abandoned/empty house: You might be ready to move on to the next phase of your life, leaving behind the house you've lived in.

Building a house: You might need to pay more attention to yourself, to "build up" some aspect of yourself that you are neglecting.

Cleaning house: You probably want or need to clear away old clutter (mental or physical) and make room for a better version of yourself.

Damaged house: A broken house in disrepair suggests that you might be ignoring some part of yourself or your unconscious mind, or perhaps you feel intruded upon, even attacked.

Haunted house: Possibly a nightmare, but also this kind of dream can indicate hidden or repressed memories and feelings, often from childhood, that still haunt you in some way.

Locked out of a house: You might fear being left out or rejected by others or by a situation. You could feel that you are no longer welcome.

Random house: Seeing any house can mean that you are thinking about yourself, since the house's rooms can represent aspects of your mind and personality.

Run-down house (1): A house that is neglected or falling down can signal the need to let go of behaviors and opinions that no longer serve you.

Run-down house (2): Alternately, a run-down house can suggest that you have aspects of your life that are cluttered, messy, and in need of repair.

Your own house: You are specifically looking at yourself, or a version of you, in the dream. You might have concerns about your home, or even a distorted view of it.

I

ICE

Dreams of ice come in several varieties, each with their own meanings:

Falling through ice: Something might be about to "crash" into your life, but it might be good (a breakthrough) or bad (an upheaval), depending on the situation.

Ice storms: Ice coming from the sky might suggest that you are feeling stuck and unable to express yourself. Perhaps you are cut off from your emotions.

Seeing ice: To see ice in some form in a dream often (though not always) refers to feeling slowed or uncertain. Ice is, of course, stilled water, and things are not flowing.

Slipping on ice: You might lack confidence and self-esteem, and could be facing obstacles on your chosen path, ones that could hurt or embarrass you.

Walking on ice: You should take extra care about a certain situation, and proceed slowly, just as you would on real ice.

INDECISION

If you cannot decide something in a dream, it more than likely means you are struggling with a similar problem in real life, which is spilling into your dream.

INSOMNIA

To dream about not being asleep might seem strange, but it often indicates that you are feeling a loss of control and need to work to regain balance in your life.

INTERVIEW

To dream of being interviewed often indicates some anxiety or a lack of confidence. You might fear being judged and worry about failing to measure up.

ISLAND

A dream of an island suggests various things, often to do with the dreamer's sense of self and relations to others:

Island (1): An island dream indicates that you are probably feeling relaxed, at ease with something in your life, perhaps as if you were on vacation.

Island (2): Alternately, an island dream might be telling you that you do need to take a vacation, reduce stress, and get away from it all.

Stranded on an island (1): Again, you might need a vacation, or you could feel disconnected from people and situations around you, and possibly even lonely.

Stranded on an island (2): Another meaning is that you might be trying to hide from problems that you would rather not face, to be a "cast-away" from your worries.

J

JAIL

If you dream about being in jail, you often feel restricted (in a job, a relationship, etc.). It might also indicate guilt over doing something wrong.

JEALOUSY

This dream might be an expression of jealous feelings you have in your life, or that you are struggling to feel worthy and might not want to get too close to someone.

JESTER

A jester in your dream can suggest that you are allowing foolish distractions to take your attention away from what you need to focus on.

JUGGLING

If you are juggling in a dream, you could be trying to take on too much all at once. If you're not careful, you're going to "drop the ball" on something.

K

KEY(S)

Keys have a lot of symbolism, so it's natural that they usually have a multitude of meanings in a dream:

Finding keys: This dream can suggest that you have found a solution to a problem, or are close to doing so. Keep looking!

Keys locking something: You might be trying to lock away something you don't wish to confront: feelings, fears, a confrontation, etc.

Keys unlocking something: You might have discovered the answer (as with finding keys), or you are about to "unlock" the next part of your life.

Losing keys: You probably fear losing something, whether it's status, control, or security, or perhaps you are experiencing unexpected changes and hardships in your life.

Sexual meanings: Dreams can have obvious sexual meanings, depending on how the key is used in the dream and whether the dream is enjoyable or unpleasant.

KING

Dreaming about a king can often symbolize a few different things:

Being the king: You have or will soon have additional power and/or authority, which is something to be proud of, but be careful not to let it go to your head.

King (1): Seeing a king can symbolize that you are successful, or will be, or hope to be. Happily, you will defeat the things standing against you.

King (2): Alternately, seeing a king can represent the need for some authority in your life, such as your father or a father figure, who can help and advise you.

KNEELING

If you are kneeling in a dream, you could be feeling submissive, or open to others' suggestions, but be careful about giving up too much of yourself to them.

KNIFE

Knives are tools, cooking implements, and weapons. How they appear in a dream will determine their possible meanings:

Attacked by a knife: If someone attacks you with a knife, you might feel threatened in your real life, especially if the attacker is someone you really know. Be careful.

Knife (1): If you are holding a knife, you might be wanting or needing to cut something or someone out of your life that no longer serves you.

Knife (2): A dream knife can also indicate sexual tension or discomfort, and you should think about what that might mean in a relationship.

Wounded by a knife: To be wounded by a knife suggests that you fear anger or aggression from someone else, whether from their temper or a physical threat. Again, be careful.

KNIGHT

To dream about a knight suggests that you value loyalty and honor, and/or you are looking for help and perhaps protection from someone. What “dragon” threatens you?

KNOT

To see a knot in a dream might indicate that you are allowing small problems to worry you too much. It can also indicate self-limiting ideas and actions.

LADDERS

Laddersare, of course, for climbing, but that can indicate many things in different dreams:

Broken ladder: You are worried about failure, and perhaps about never getting the chance to "climb" the way you would like.

Falling from a ladder: You might be fearing taking a risk, or you fear the consequences of trying something new, even getting hurt in the process.

Holding onto a ladder: If you or someone is holding a ladder, it can mean that you have the support system around you to help you succeed, or that you enjoy helping others.

Ladder (1): You are mindful of the work you have put in to achieve your goals. Things are paying off (or soon will), and you are climbing.

Ladder (2): You might be embarking on a new journey in life, perhaps a spiritual one, and are beginning to see your life in new and different ways.

Walking under a ladder: Of course, we associate this with back luck, but in a dream, it could mean that you are regretting a decision, or fearing the outcome of it.

LATENESS

No one really likes being late, even though it happens to the best of us. It can also happen in our dreams:

Being late (1): You might be afraid of change and are seeking some way of putting it off. If you can be late in your unconscious mind, that change might not happen.

Being late (2): You could possibly be afraid of making a difficult choice and are delaying it until you can get more clarification, or maybe you're procrastinating about it.

Being late (3): You might fear that you are running out of time to do everything that you want to do, that time is slipping away.

Being late (4): Alternately, being late in your dream might be your way of telling yourself that it will be okay anyway: "better late than never."

LAUGHTER

Laughter can have more than one meaning in a dream, and not always for the good:

Being laughed at: You might feel insecure or inadequate, or that no matter what you do, people will laugh at you and not take you seriously.

Laughing (1): You are likely experiencing happiness or amusement in your life about something, or perhaps you need to. What could bring laughter into your life?

Laughing (2): Alternately, you might or might not be happy. Laughing can be a sign of a need to loosen up, and not take things to heart so much.

Mocking laughter: If you hear laughter that is mocking or "evil," it suggests that you are feeling conspired against, or that you think your situation is hopeless.

LETTERS OF THE ALPHABET

Letters of the alphabet in a dream can stand for anything that letter spells. A "j" might mean someone is looking for a new job, for example. Analyze these letters carefully.

LIGHT

Most would interpret light in a dream as a positive sign, representing knowledge illumination, hope, and so on. Here are some specific meanings:

Bright light: An especially bright light could be drawing your attention to something important, showing you the way to new insights and enlightenment.

Light (1): Seeing a light often means "seeing the light," i.e., gaining understanding or insights into a situation, a problem, etc., that has been eluding you.

Light (2): You might be finally getting the truth about something that has been obscured until now. This can be good or bad, depending on the situation.

Light bulb: You might have a new idea, or you might be ready to accept something in your life for what it really is, rather than what you want it to be.

Soft light: Your unconscious mind might be trying to communicate with you in some way. What are you feeling about a situation that needs more examination?

Unable to turn on a light: If you are trying to find a light switch or otherwise illuminate an area, you are probably lacking sufficient information about something to see it clearly.

LIGHTHOUSE

A lighthouse in your dream can suggest that you are in need of assistance while facing a difficult situation. You might feel adrift and need advice.

LIST

If you are making a list in your dream, you are trying to get organized, and might be worried about something in your life that needs to be set in order.

LOST

A dream of being lost is common, and usually indicates that the dreamer is struggling with something:

Lost and late for something: Your probably feel unprepared or distracted and unable to meet your obligations for something in your waking life.

Needing to get home: This dream suggests that you feel unsafe or out of your comfort zone about something and want to find your way back to safety.

Unfamiliar surroundings: Being lost in a new neighborhood or city can mean the need for more information about a project, relationship, situation, or anything that you are invested in.

Wandering while lost: You might be trying to figure out something important, but maybe you don't have all the necessary information yet. The path forward is not known.

M

MAP

Reading a map indicates that you are on the right path in your life. If you can't understand the map, you might be feeling lost and in need of aid for your life's direction.

MASK

Masks hide things of course, and such a dream might be reflecting that in different ways:

COVID-19 mask: If you are wearing a protective mask, or perhaps not wearing one, in a crowded area, it could suggest that you are feeling vulnerable to outside attacks and/or influences.

Removing a mask (1): If you remove a mask you are wearing, you might be ready to share more about yourself, or finally tell the truth about something.

Removing a mask (2): If someone else removes their mask, perhaps you now see them differently than you did before, which might be good or bad.

Seeing someone in a mask: You might have trouble trusting people, or one person in particular. You might fear they are hiding something, lying to you, or maybe you envy them.

Wearing a mask (1): You are probably hiding some aspect of yourself or your feelings from others. You might fear that they won't like you if they see the "real" you.

Wearing a mask (2): You could be having conflict with someone over a miscommunication or misunderstanding. What are you hiding from each other?

MAZE

Seeing a maze might indicate that you are lost, confused, and/or need a new direction, or that you need to make things easier and take a more direct approach to something.

MEDIEVAL

If you dream of medieval times, you might be nostalgic or longing for something now gone, or you might have some outdated ideas that need to be refreshed.

MILK

Milk can have multiple meanings in a dream, depending on the situation:

Drinking milk: If you are drinking milk, you are probably happy with your home life, and/or you want (or perhaps need) to improve your relationships with others.

Hot milk: Hot milk suggests home, rest, comfort, and serenity. Just as you might take some before bed to help you sleep, you are feeling relaxed.

Seeing milk: Milk in a dream can mean maternal love, or caring and compassion from anyone. You either have or want these feelings in your life.

Sour milk: You might need to stand back for a while and be more observant, as you might be trusting a person or situation too much, which could be a bad idea.

Spilled milk: Spilled milk often represents that you are losing your trust in a person or situation, or that you have lost a chance to do something you wanted to do.

MIST

A dream of mist, or being in a mist points to you being uncertain, even confused about something your life. You need more clarification to part the mists around you.

MONEY

For better or worse, money is an important part of most people's lives, so it's only natural that we dream about it for different reasons:

Abundant money: If positive, it could indicate that money is coming into your life, but if negative, it could mean the opposite, or refer to your fears about financial loss.

Asking/begging for money: You might be feeling anxious or fearful about your financial situation, or you might think that you need to rely on other people too much.

Borrowing money: You could be facing uncertainty about the future, and feeling powerless to do what you need or want to do without significant help, or difficult decisions.

Coins: A dream about coins might suggest that you're making slow but steady progress, or acquiring what you want and need in small but measurable amounts.

Credit Cards: You might worry about owing others, about being in their debt in some way, or perhaps you are expecting too much of them or yourself.

Finding money: If you find money in a dream, you are probably feeling secure about your life, your finances, and your direction, or you might soon bring in more money.

Having no money: If you have no money, you probably fear that you don't have the resources to make your goals a reality, whether that's financial, new skills, or circumstances.

Hoarding money: If you dream about hoarding money, you could be feeling insecure about something that you want to hang on to, or even selfish about it.

Lending money: You might have a need to be more helpful and charitable, whether to a specific person (if you know the person in the dream), or to society (if you don't).

Losing your money: You might be feeling a lack of control, or even self-esteem. You could also fear being trapped in a situation and not having a way to get out.

Paper money: Paper money is tangible, but fragile. Are you worried about not being able to hold onto it? Are there things you can do to bring more money into your life?

Receiving an incorrect amount of money: You could worry that a person or situation is "short-changing" you, or maybe that you don't deserve anything better.

Spending money: Spending can suggest that you are generous, or perhaps that you are looking for a romantic relationship. If you are not single, you might want to rekindle the romance.

Stealing money: You might need to be more cautious about your behavior, or this dream could mean that you need more love, or to be careful in your ambitions.

Stolen money: You are possibly being taken advantage of in some situation, or by a specific person, and you should consider taking extra precautions to protect yourself.

Winning money/the lottery: You probably desire to be rewarded for your efforts, and to become more secure in your life. Or perhaps you are open to new gifts.

MONTHS OF THE YEAR

Dreams can incorporate the different months as background settings, and often the weather associated with them, to mean different things:

January: A dream about January can indicate that you have lost, or fear losing, someone you love, and all that goes with that.

February: Surprisingly, dreams about this month can often indicate sadness and poor health, and perhaps the desire to be whole and loved. Valentine's Day is only one day of the month!

March: March dreams sometimes point to disappointments in your life, though often with the promise of new beginnings to follow, if you persevere.

April: You might be about to receive a reward of some kind, though an April Fool's Day dream might simply be telling you that you are acting foolish.

May: Good times are in store for you, or are already happening. But the dream might also signify that you are asking for permission about something: "may" I?

June: If you dream of June, you might be seeing (or hoping to see) progress in the projects you've been working on. This could include a promotion, financial gain, and more.

July: Dreaming of July might indicate that you are feeling hopeful about a project or the future, and being productive enough to take it on.

August: You might be dealing with some kind of miscommunication or lack of understanding in your work or personal life, something that needs to be cleared up.

September: September in a dream generally means good luck, or at least that you desire to have good luck in the waking world, especially if you've been feeling unlucky.

October: You are enjoying (or will soon enjoy) success for all of your hard work, and bringing in the "fruits of your labor."

November: You might be acting oblivious to, or at least unbothered by, some problem in your life. You will need to determine if this is a wise course of action or not.

December: This month can signify happy gatherings and friendships for you, or at least your longing to have these in your life. Also, it indicates gifts and a giving nature.

MOON

Moon dreams can be as mysterious as they seem:

Blood moon: A red or "blood" moon can suggest upcoming challenges and changes, often involving endings and/or difficulties. Repressed feelings can also be indicated.

Crescent moon: A crescent moon or new moon often symbolizes potential new beginnings, usually for the better, and it confirms that you are on the right path.

Eclipse: You might be hiding something from your-self (often your more feminine side and attributes), or perhaps that side is about to be revealed.

Full moon: Something is being completed, or will be, and you are more deeply connected with your spiritual side at this time.

Multiple moons: Many moons can indicate confusion and turmoil, but also deep intuition and the need to follow it and connect more deeply with your feminine side.

Two moons: Dreaming of two moons sometimes communicates that you are being pulled in different directions, possibly by opposing forces in your life.

MUD

A dream about mud usually indicates a negative in a dreamer's life:

Mud on clothing or your body: You might feel attacked, ganged-up on, or even the subject of unfair slander. You may have to defend yourself.

Seeing mud: You are likely dealing with a "messy" problem in your life, probably one that is going to require a lot of "clean up" to fix.

Walking in mud: If you are stepping in mud, you might feel stuck or frustrated in your situation, whether it be your work, a friendship, your love life, or something else.

MUSIC

Music features commonly in dreams, and given the infinite variety of musical styles in the world, it's not possible to list them all, but here are some common ones:

Blues: You could be experiencing something in your waking life that is making you sad and/or regretful. Perhaps you've lost something and can't get it back.

Classical: You possibly yearn for greater peace in your life, or perhaps you desire more elegance and refinement, or a return to something older and more established.

Country: Is there something from your past that you are longing for or trying to recapture? Did it leave you unexpectedly?

Dance music: You might need to express yourself more, to let it all hang out. You could be feeling frustrated about not being able to be freer with yourself.

Heavy Metal: You could have pent up aggressions and anger that need to be let out in a healthy way. These feelings can be positive if channeled correctly.

Folk: You could be feeling the need to connect (or reconnect) with your heritage, especially if the music is a part of your own cultural background.

Gospel: This dream might have to do with your spiritual beliefs, or it could be that you are feeling filled with hope and faith of any kind.

Jazz: You might be excited about an upcoming project, especially if you have the freedom to really delve into it with your own unique ideas.

Latin: Latin music is often energetic and joyful, so perhaps you are ready to let your hair down and party! How might being less inhibited work for you?

Music in general (1): If you like the musical genre you are dreaming, it can indicate happiness and contentment, paying attention to any specific meanings listed here.

Music in general (2): Alternately, if you don't like the style of music in your dream, you could interpret these meanings in the opposite way, or maybe you're ignoring them.

New Age: You probably desire peace and tranquility in your life, or need to work on surrounding yourself with these things. This dream can also indicate spiritual needs.

Pop: This dream might speak to your sense of fun and recapturing that if it is missing in your life. If it's music you enjoy, how do you feel when listening to it?

Rap: If you hear rap or are doing the rapping, it could be that you need to speak out more and communicate your ideas and thoughts to others more clearly.

Rock: You might be feeling a lack of excitement in your life, and/or wanting others to look up to you, to be your "fans."

Soul: You could be experiencing nostalgia for an earlier time, especially if you lived through it, and perhaps you are committed to social issues, both now and in the past.

World: Music from a specific part of the world could represent your attachment to that place and culture, or perhaps your desire to visit, if you don't already live there.

MUSICAL INSTRUMENTS

There are thousands of different musical instruments in the world, but here are some of the one you are probably most familiar with and likely to encounter in your dreams:

Bass: You are feeling (or hoping to feel) in sync with everything around you, but you might also feel that you are not valued enough by others.

Cello: You are probably proud of something you have recently accomplished and want to share it. This can be creative, work-related, or even sensual in nature.

Drums: You "march to your own drum beat," and stand by your decisions. You are likely making regular progress toward your goals at an even pace.

Flute: Flutes often indicate smooth sailing, but they can also point to loss and a longing for something. They can also be phallic symbols related to these options.

Guitar: If you see or are playing a guitar, it can be a symbol of your creativity and need for expression (artistic or otherwise), and it can also indicate sexual desire.

Harp: A harp can stand for harmony and healing. You might be experiencing either of these in your life, or you need to in some way.

Horn: It is probably time for you to pay closer attention to your inner thoughts, and also be mindful if you are bragging about anything.

Lute: A lute can represent your faith in yourself or in something in your life. It might be something that you value highly, a precious item worthy of admiration.

Organ: Dreaming about an organ (such as a pipe organ) can be a commentary on your spiritual and/or religious beliefs, or lack thereof, and how you view those.

Piano: You are probably feeling happy with things in your life right now, though if you're playing the piano, you might still be searching for that satisfaction.

Synthesizer: You might need to adopt new methods and ideas in your work or personal life, to "synthesize" the new and the old to create something better.

Trombone: The trombone can mean that you are doing well in your romantic life, or that you will be in the near future. Keep doing what you're doing!

Trumpet: You might need to pay closer attention to something in your life that is potentially a problem, even dangerous. Look around for warning signs.

Violin: The violin often represents culture and harmony in one's life, and the desire for those things. Playing the violin suggests that you are recognized and appreciated for your work.

N

NAKED

Another common dream (like being in one's underwear) that suggests various vulnerabilities and is not always sexual:

Everyone else is naked: If you are the only one clothed, you might be concealing something, or you worry about standing out; you might also be overly critical of others.

Naked in public (1): To be naked in public conveys that you might be afraid of being discovered for something you've done in secret, or that you're being judged.

Naked in public (2): You might feel unprepared for some situation, and/or fearful that everyone will see you as you truly are, that you'll be exposed.

Someone else is naked (1): If you see someone else naked and enjoy the sight, you might be very accepting and open minded, or else you might think that you "see through" the person.

Someone else is naked (2): If you see someone naked and don't enjoy the sight, you might be unhappy to discover the truth about someone or about a situation you're dealing with.

Suddenly naked: If you suddenly lose all your clothes, it might indicate that you feel exposed and want to cover up something about yourself or a situation.

NATURAL DISASTERS

Natural disasters can take many terrifying forms, both in the waking world and in dreams:

Asteroid: To dream of an asteroid impact suggests that you are experiencing something that is "shattering" your world: a belief, an ideal, or perhaps a feeling of assuredness.

Avalanche: Dreaming of an avalanche or mudslide indicates that you might be keeping emotions or thoughts pent up, and that these need release and to be dealt with.

Earthquake: Something in your life might have been shaken up, whether a relationship, a job, a family situation, etc., and you no longer feel fully in control.

Floods: Some emotions can no longer be contained, and you cannot hold them back, but unleashing them could bring disaster on those around you.

Hurricane: You might fear an attack from some outside force, whether it be on your home, yourself, loved ones, or anything else that might be important to you.

Tidal wave: As with flooding, you could be repressing feelings or holding something back that is threatening to overwhelm you. Letting it out is necessary, but potentially dangerous.

Tornado: Stress, anger, and emotional turmoil might be threatening you in your life, whether now or in the near future. You need to brace yourself for what's coming.

Volcano: You might have repressed anger and stress that are "bubbling up," threatening to erupt and unleash damage on those around you. Be careful.

Wildfire: You could be struggling to control your feelings about something, and these thoughts are threatening to get away from you (see "Fire" for other possible options).

NATURE

Being out in nature in a dream can speak to your need for beauty, solitude, connection to the world, and rejuvenating yourself. You might simply need to experience it more.

NAUSEA

To dream of being nauseated can mean that you are facing some negative issue in your life that they need to be rid of, to purge.

NET

To dream of a net might indicate that you feel trapped in some situation. On the other hand, it might be telling you to "cast your net" out to new opportunities and contacts.

NIGHTMARE

Everyone has nightmares occasionally, and they are often negative or inverted versions of many other entries in this dictionary. So, consult specific topics to see what your nightmare might be telling you.

NO

Saying "no" in your dream often means that you are doing so in your waking life, and standing up for yourself, or perhaps you need to, even if you risk unpopularity.

NOSTALGIA

A nostalgia dream might mean that you are longing for something simpler or comforting, or a return to a happier time, such as childhood. You want things to be easier.

NUMBERS

Of course, numbers are infinite, and we cannot hope to include all possibilities, but here is a list of some common dream numbers and their potential meanings:

0: You might be feeling empty, or perhaps there is a void in your life that you cannot fill. Or, you might feel that you are going in circles.

1: You could be feeling like "number one" at the moment, at the top of your game and in a position of power, but it might also symbolize being alone or loneliness.

2: This number can symbolize partnerships, duality, the need for balance in your life, and things like marriages or cooperation, depending on your situation.

3: This dream might refer to past, present, and future, or to mind, body, and spirit, or any situation where three is a vital number.

4: You might be thinking about stability (four corners), or material goods. In some Asian cultures, the number actually represents death.

5: This number can mean the five senses, and perhaps your need to be better attuned to them and your surroundings. Are things working for you the way you want?

6: Often a number of harmony and peace, it can represent comfort, love, familial connections, and happiness, or the feeling of balance in your own life.

7: There are many different sevens (days, sins, chakras, and more), so your "seven" dream might be your thoughts on any of these, or your desire to be unique.

8: This dream might be telling you to trust your gut about something, especially if it will lead to greater success and the rewards that you feel you are due.

9: Things are coming to a head, and completion is near. You are doing the right things, taking the correct actions, and are in it for the long haul.

10: As with nine, you are completing something, but also possibly about to start something new. The number can also represent law and order.

20: You are probably seeing things more clearly now (think 20/20 vision), but you still might need help in addressing the situation.

25: You might be dwelling on something that is no longer serving any purpose. It's probably time to move on and seek something new.

50: A celebration might be at hand, but it also might indicate that you need to share something (think 50/50), or even that you are entitled to your fair share.

100: You might need to "give it 100%" in some situation in your waking life. Maybe you've been holding back, but now isn't the time to do that.

1,000: You might be about to begin a new time of growth and potential transformation, which can include new insights, new spiritual realizations, or personal development.

Dates: If you dream about a date that is significant to you (say, a birthday), it could indicate coming success. If you can remember the date, look it up when you can.

Even numbers: Viewing even numbers can mean that you are feeling balanced in your life, happy and at peace. Or perhaps you want these feelings.

Lottery numbers: Though these numbers might not help you win the actual lottery (sorry!), a dream of such a win can indicate that success is on the way in some form.

Multiple numbers: Any combination of numbers might indicate that you should look at each and combine their meanings, e.g., 23, 47, 368, etc.

Numbers in the sky: Numbers hovering in the sky in your dream might be your mind's way of telling you that you are working too hard and need a break.

Odd numbers: Seeing multiple odd numbers in a dream can mean that you could be wrestling with an unresolved situation or feelings, perhaps of anger.

Repeating numbers: Dreams about a number that repeats (say, 444) might have special significance, and you should consider them in light of their various individual meanings.

O

OFFICE

Offices can intrude into dreams, and often have work-related meanings:

Your own office: You might be proud of your accomplishments, but you also could be struggling with work/life balance, and need to adjust.

Someone else's office: If you are in another office (or one you don't recognize), perhaps you are trying too hard to compare yourself to others.

OPERATION

If you don't have a procedure scheduled in reality, this dream may indicate feelings of vulnerability and openness to change coming into your life.

OUTSIDE

Dreaming of being outside often represents a feeling of freedom and possibilities, or perhaps the need to break free and not limit yourself to a metaphorical inside.

OVEN

We associate ovens with cooking, but dreams sometimes have different ideas:

Oven (1): Ovens represent food, warmth, sharing, and good company. You are probably either grateful for these things in your life, or want more of them.

Oven (2): This might speak to your or desire, or fear, about having children. How you react to the oven in your dream will help you understand your feelings better.

P

PACKAGE

A package in the mail is something we usually like to get, and often means one of two things in a dream:

Receiving a package: You are bringing new assets into your life that you need, or perhaps you are learning new things that will bring about success.

Sending a package: You might be offloading your problems, feelings, etc., onto someone else, instead of confronting them yourself. Be careful about what you give away.

PARALYZED

Dreaming of being paralyzed can be disorienting, even frightening. Depending on the context, it can mean different things:

Paralyzed (1): In REM sleep, our brain immobilizes our bodies to prevent us from moving. Waking abruptly can sometimes mean the brain and body have to "catch up" and we briefly can't move. Breathe and wait.

Paralyzed (2): Feeling paralyzed in a dream can indicate that you feel powerless or helpless about something, unable to take action. What can you do to "unstick" yourself?

Paralyzed (3): You might also be wrestling with your feelings about something or someone, and can't express them properly; this is the feeling of being stuck or immobile.

PARANOID

If you are paranoid in your dream, you might be feeling hesitant about taking the next step in a relationship, a career, or some other situation. Maybe you can't do it yet.

PARTIES/GATHERINGS

Party dreams are fairly common, or any gatherings where people socialize and eat or drink. Here are some indications of what they might mean:

Alone at a party: If you are alone, or surrounded by people you don't know, you might be feeling isolated, or in need of new or more (or better?) friends.

Birthday party: Dreaming about your birthday party can mean that you are happy with the social life you have and feel appreciated by those around you.

Enjoying a party: This dream might be telling you to get out more, to mingle with others, and put yourself forward in social situations.

Invited to a party: You could be enjoying the support of others right now or wanting to. Or, perhaps you feel left out and want to be included.

Not enjoying a party: If you don't like the party, you are probably annoyed by someone (or several people) in your life right now and want to be left alone.

Planning a party: Perhaps you are overthinking something, especially if it's for fun. Or, you might need extra help in preparing, especially if it's recreational.

PERFUME

Wearing perfume in a dream can symbolize a desire for more luxury and pleasure, while smelling it can mean that you have nostalgia for something in your past.

PHONE

Our phones often dominate our lives, for better and worse, so it's only natural that they will show up in dreams in a number of different ways, often involving communication:

Missed phone call: There might be a miscommunication with someone in your life. Alternately, you might be worried about a friend or a family member.

Phone (1): A phone can indicate the way in which you communicate with others, whether easily or with more difficulties. Consider the context.

Phone (2): It's possible that you need to improve your communication skills all around, or that you need to face up to something you've been putting off.

Phone call from a friend: You might be hoping to hear from this person, or you might need to reach out to them. There could also be an issue that you two need to resolve.

Phone call from a stranger: Be careful not to alienate others in your interactions with them. You might not be communicating well with them at this time.

Phone call on hold: You might feel constrained from being yourself, or you fear that others are relying on you too much, even taking you for granted.

Phone number: You probably need to reach out to someone in your life. You might need their assistance, or they might need yours.

Phone number (unable to remember): It's possible that you are relying too much on others for help, support, etc., and you need to be more independent.

Phone ringing: You could be having issues with communicating with others in your waking life. They are trying to get through to you, but you are not "answering."

Texting: Texting in general often refers to how you relate to your friends and family. It might be easier for you to put something in writing than to say it out loud.

Receiving a text: Someone might be trying to reach out to you to offer help or advice. This person could be a friend or they will become one.

Wrong number: If you dial a wrong number, you might be having trouble expressing yourself clearly to someone, or perhaps you don't understand each other.

PILL

To take a pill in a dream might mean that you are trying to heal yourself, or you might be facing up to something you don't like, the proverbial "bitter pill to swallow."

POINTING

Pointing in a dream will probably mean one of two things, depending on the pointer:

Someone points at you: You might be feeling guilty about something you've done, or fearing that others are accusing you of doing something wrong.

You are pointing: You need to pay attention to whatever you're pointing at (the thing or person). Or, a solution you need to a problem could be right in front of you.

POLE

Seeing a pole in your dream can mean that you have things in your life you can rely on and that give you stability. Or, it can be a phallic symbol!

PSYCHIC DREAMS

Psychic dreams are controversial, with many people not accepting that they exist at all. Here is a guide to different types you might have, if you believe that they are real. Be sure to write them down as soon as you can:

Being psychic in a dream: You might have a well-developed sense of your insights and intuitions. If you get psychic impressions along with this dream, definitely pay attention to them.

Clairvoyant dreams: You might be picking up information about something happening in the moment, perhaps far away from you. Follow up as soon as you can to verify your dream.

Dreams about the dead: Some believe that being visited by a dead person in a dream really is that person's spirit reaching out to you. Pay close attention to what they say.

Intuition: Your unconscious might be trying to confirm something in your waking life that you have a strong feeling about. Pay attention to what your intuition is telling you.

Precognition: Precognitive dreams usually present you with symbols and sensations, rather than concrete images, but they can tell you a lot about a situation.

Premonition: Premonitions are often images or feelings about something that hasn't happened yet. If you feel strongly about it, keep an eye on what occurs in the coming days and weeks.

Psychokinesis/telekinesis: If you dream that you can move objects with your mind, you might need to ease up on your need to control things in your waking life.

Seeing a psychic: If you dream about seeing a psychic, you could be searching for answers to a troubling problem, seeking advice on how to handle it. You might also fear failure.

Telepathic dreams (1): You might have a dream that gives you some insight into another's thoughts or their state (health, mental wellbeing, life status, etc.). Check in with them if it feels appropriate.

Telepathic dreams (2): Alternately, having a dream about being a telepath might mean that you need to pay more attention to what those around youare saying.

PUBLIC SPEAKING

A dream about being in front of an audience and speaking, or perhaps performing music or some other art form can mean any of the following:

Audience ignores you: This kind of dream indicates that you might feel unacknowledged, unimportant, or not taken seriously in your waking life.

Being unprepared to speak: Being unready to speak or perform suggests anxiety, whether about an actual upcoming speech, or of being ridiculed or failing in your life in general.

Listening to a speaker: This dream can mean the dreamer wants to be heard, or to express themselves to others in new or important ways.

Speaking to an audience: If the person dreams of speaking without fear, it might indicate that they feel the need to communicate better in their lives or give important news.

Q

QUEEN

A dream of a queen often represents a maternal figure in your life, or feelings of power and influence (whether you already have those qualities or want them).

QUESTION

Asking a question in a dream can point to your ignorance about a subject, or your self-doubt in dealing with something. Do you remember what you asked?

QUIET

If it is very quiet in your dream, then you might be seeking this peace in your waking life. You need to slow down and go inward.

R

RAIN

Dreaming of rain can indicate tears or sadness, but also relief, and the sense of being cleansed and letting something go, and perhaps forgiveness.

RAINBOW

Rainbows can appear in dreams in a variety of ways, both natural and "unnatural." Here are some of their meanings:

Rainbow: Generally, rainbows can indicate good fortune, success, money (think of the pot of gold), and leaving your troubles in the past, or hoping to.

Rainbow at night: A rainbow at night could symbolize your connection with your unconscious, or your desire to be better in touch with it and your emotions.

Rainbow bridge: You might wish for, or have recently created, a bridge between two parts of your life that you want connected.

Rainbow colors: Seeing something in rainbow colors might be telling you that you need to look at a person or a situation in a more positive way, and maybe be more hopeful.

Rainbow inside: You might be undergoing some important internal growth and changes, especially if the rainbow is inside your home.

Rainbow hair: This dream speaks to your overall nature and suggests that you are moving in the right direction. Like the hair, you are growing and vibrant.

Upside down rainbow: Important things might be about to change in your life, probably for the better. Something is about to "turn up."

REACHING

If you are reaching for something in your dream, you probably want something you don't have yet, whether it's money, career, love, or emotional contentment.

READING

Reading something in a dream often indicates that you are seeking more information or knowledge, especially if you don't understand the words. You need to think things through more.

RECURRING DREAMS

Almost everyone has recurring dreams, which can be about any of the entries in this dictionary. They often indicate unresolved problems or emotions, or perhaps unmet needs. Combine these meanings with any entry here to gain more insight into yours.

REGRET

You are probably feeling regret about something in your waking life, but you might not have expressed it yet, or you might be disappointed in something, even yourself.

RELIEF

To dream of relief suggests that you want to be free of something that is troubling you, whether it's work or personal. Or, you must let go of a bigger burden.

RETREATING

If you are retreating from something, you probably don't yet have the ability to face a similar challenge in your life. Regroup and try again.

RIVER

Rivers often occur in dreams where you are trying to get somewhere, or are feeling swept up in daily life. Here are some possible meanings:

Crossing a river: You probably need to confront something that is hindering your progress, and you will have to figure out how to get past it to move on.

Dirty river: If there is dirt or mud in the river, you might need more clarity before making a decision, or you might feel that you are not settled.

Overflowing river: The pressures of life are probably getting to you, and you fear being overwhelmed, even consumed. It's time to take a step back.

River (1): You are perhaps letting life flow by a little too much. You might need to be less passive and take more control over your direction.

River (2): You might be recognizing that life is in a constant state of change and that you cannot "cross the same river twice," as the ancient Greek philosophers would say.

River (3): You could be seeking a deeper connection between your conscious and unconscious mind, or perhaps to gain a better handle on your emotions.

Raging river (1): Life is probably presenting you with challenges beyond the usual ups and downs, but you are feeling ready to take them on, to "ride the rapids."

Raging river (2): Alternately, you might be feeling as if you are being swept away, perhaps emotionally or career-wise, and you're trying hard to get your bearings.

Swimming in a river: You are likely going with the flow, but in a good way, one that is allowing you to navigate the turbulence and stay on top.

ROAD

Seeing a road in a dream often refers to your perceived direction in life, but will mean different things according to your situation and the type of dream:

Blocked road: Perhaps obviously, you have encountered some roadblocks in your waking life that you will have to navigate and work to clear, whether personal or professional.

Darkened road: You might need to make a decision on something that you are unsure about, such as taking a leap of faith or a "stab in the dark."

Dirt road: Your goals will take hard work on your part, if you want to "pave the road" and reach them. This dream reflects the efforts you need to make.

Paved road: You have already laid down the foundations of the work needed to succeed and are now traveling along the path. Keep on paving!

Road signs: Can you read what the road sign is saying? It might be an important message from your unconscious mind about what you need to do next.

Roadkill: A dead animal on the road often indicates that something is dying in your life, most often metaphorically: a job, a relationship, or a way of thinking or being.

Roadwork: Roadwork often represents the obstacles you encounter in your life in trying to get to where you want to go. Your journey might take longer than you want or expect.

Straight road: You are proceeding ahead in the way that you want, and you should not face too many obstacles on the way to success.

Unfamiliar road: You might be setting out in new and unknown directions, and be afraid of that. Trust that this road will take you where you want to go.

Winding road: You might be experiencing difficulties and setbacks in your life right now, and will have to navigate them slowly and carefully to get past them.

S

SADNESS

Dreaming about being sad very likely indicates that you feel sad about something or someone in your waking life. It can also suggest that it's time to try to let the sadness go, if you can.

SEARCHING

Searching for something in a dream indicates that there is something in your life that you need and have yet to find, whether it's love, career satisfaction, more friends, and so on.

SEXUAL DREAMS

Sexual dreams can have a variety of meanings beyond the obvious, but of course, they can also indicate exactly what you think they do:

Bisexual sex: You might be experiencing some confusion or repression about something in your life. If you are bisexual, it can be a confirmation of being comfortable with yourself.

Homosexual sex: If you are heterosexual, you could want or need to have more self-acceptance. If you are homosexual, it is likely an expression of your identity and needs.

Masturbation: You might be craving more independence, or have a need to "take matters into your own hands," when pursuing your happiness and goals.

Orgasming: Orgasming in a dream obviously has a sexual component, but it could also mean that you no longer can hold yourself back, that you need to let something out.

Sex denied: You might be wrestling with feeling unworthy, unattractive, or unwanted, whether in a current relationship or some other situation. It might be time to talk about it.

Sex in public: You could be craving attention, recognition, or the need to try something new. Or, you worry that others are talking about your sex life.

Sex tape: If you dream about being filmed having sex, then you are probably comfortable with yourself in many ways, and open to exposing yourself more.

Sex toys: You might be feeling dissatisfied with something (not necessarily your sex life), and are looking for something to make it more interesting.

Sex with a celebrity: You probably want more recognition in your life, and to be more successful in your work or other pursuits.

Sex with a co-worker: You probably don't want to have sex with them (don't worry!), but there might be something about them that you admire and wish you could emulate.

Sex with a friend (1): This dream might simply indicate that you and your friend are close and can trust each other, not necessarily that you actually want to have sex with them.

Sex with a friend (2): Of course, this dream might be telling you that you are attracted to your friend, but don't know how to approach them about the subject. Tread carefully!

Sex with multiple partners: You could be experiencing feelings of detachment in a relationship of some kind and are looking for ways to make up for that.

Sex with a monster or alien: You could harbor a desire to explore something new (maybe even taboo) sexually speaking, or you want to examine your own sexual desires and urges.

Sex with a non-partner: This dream doesn't necessarily mean you want to cheat. You might feel inhibited, or in a rut, and have the need to spice things up a bit.

Sex with a stranger (1): You might be feeling uncertain about something important in your life, or a future event that is coming toward you.

Sex with a stranger (2): This dream could also be a sign that you are more open to taking chances and being uninhibited in your dealings with others.

Sex with an authority figure: Sex with a powerful figure, such as a boss, can relate to your own need to be in control, or to be mindful of your connections to those with power.

Sex with an ex: You might be hanging onto the past too much, or maybe you keep looking for the same kind of person as a romantic partner.

Sex with your partner: This is often a fairly straightforward dream that simply means you desire your partner and that desire flows over into your dreams. Enjoy!

Sexual dream (1): Your mind might be telling you that you need better (or more) sexual outlets for yourself in the way that works best for you.

Sexual dream (2): Perhaps you are trying to become more whole in mind and body and the partner in your dream represents those qualities you would like more of.

Sexual dream (3): You could be craving more intimacy in an existing relationship, or need to express your feelings to your partner clearly and more often.

Watching a partner have sex: This dream suggests that you are more passive in your relationship, and perhaps you worry that you cannot satisfy your partner.

Watching others have sex: You perhaps need to be more adventurous in your life and your sex life. Consider "getting off the sidelines" and participating more.

SHAPE-SHIFTING/MORPHING

Dreams about a metamorphosis most often indicate change in your life, in a variety of ways:

Object shifting (1): To see something change into something else suggests a change is coming in your life. Also, you might need to change how you are looking at something.

Object shifting (2): Alternately, this dream can indicate that you are having a difficult time making up your mind about something, or are weighing the options.

Shifting into an animal: If you find yourself turning into an animal in a dream, you might be feeling constrained and want to let out your inner wild side.

Shifting into someone else (1): It's possible that you just need to start viewing things from another person's point of view, to get inside their head.

Shifting into someone else (2): You might need to incorporate qualities from someone you know into your own life, basically to be more like them.

SINKING

If you are sinking into the ground, you probably feel insecure or even betrayed. You thought someone or something had a more solid basis, and trusted them too much.

SKYSCRAPER

You probably have big ideas and goals, or high-minded ideals and creative talents. If you recognize the skyscraper, this dream may have additional personal meaning for you.

SLOW MOTION

If you are moving slowly, like time has been slowed down, you are probably frustrated or thwarted, feeling like something is taking too long, which is stressful.

SNAKE

Snakes often bring about negative reactions from people, but their dream meanings are many:

Chased by a snake: You could be avoiding something, maybe deliberately, and you might fear having to confront it. This may be a part of yourself that you don't want to face.

Dead snake: You might be grateful that something threatening to you has passed or maybe your mind is telling you there is nothing more to fear.

Eaten by a snake: You might fear that a person or situation is taking advantage of you, controlling you, or causing you to disappear.

General dream about a snake: If the snake presents no danger, the dream can often refer to the melding of the conscious and unconscious minds.

Killing a snake: You might be conquering some obstacle, overcoming a fear, having revenge, or ridding yourself of a danger.

Multiple snakes: You could be about to undergo some major shifts and changes in your life, or you might be feeling overwhelmed.

Snake bite (1): You might be feeling the need to protect yourself from someone or a certain situation, and you probably need to be careful in dealing with them.

Snake bite (2): If the snake is venomous, it can indicate some danger (real or imagined) that you must contend with, or you have fears that you must deal with.

Snake bite (3): The dream might be a warning not to be tempted too much by someone or a situation that seems appealing, because they might ultimately prove to be dangerous.

Snake in your house: Something might be entering into your mind, for good or ill, depending on how the snake is perceived in the dream.

Snake on the bed: You might have some anxiety around your sexuality or a partner's. Perhaps your partner intimidates you in some way, or you feel inadequate.

Two-headed snake: This dream can indicate that you are being pulled in opposite directions, especially if the two heads are on opposite sides of the snake's body.

SPIDER

Spiders are nightmare fuel for many, but their presence in dreams can contain many different meanings, scary and not so scary:

Chased by one or more spiders: You might fear being overwhelmed by something, especially a maternal figure or even your own emotions, or getting trapped in a situation.

Killing a spider: You might be seeking to escape from something to save yourself, but you might also be killing your feminine side or intuition. Pay closer attention.

Spider bites: This dream can mean that unconscious emotions are bubbling up, or perhaps that you are having conflicts with a maternal figure.

Spider on the bed: This dream might indicate intimacy issues, or the desire to explore something more intimate, depending on whether you react positively or negatively to the spider.

Spiderwebs: A web can represent several different parts of your life, and how you are reacting to them. Or it might mean that you want to attract someone or something.

Surrounded by spiders: You might feel that you are being attacked, even ganged-up on, or that something in your life is beyond your control.

Walking into spiderwebs: If webs cling to you, it can mean that there are parts of your life and psyche that you are ignoring, ones that will "stick" until you address them.

SPRING

A dream about the season of spring shows that you are likely feeling hopeful, optimistic, and seeking out new possibilities and opportunities.

SUMMER

Dreaming about summer suggests that you are hopeful, optimistic about growth and new opportunities, learning new things, and perhaps expanding who you are.

SURPRISE

If you are surprised in a dream, you might be feeling unready for a situation, or alternately that you need a new challenge or task, something that will surprise you.

SURREAL DREAMS

We've all had dreams that are bizarre, fantastical, or just don't make sense. There are many possible meanings for them; here are a few:

Surreal (1): You might need to break away from rational thinking for a bit and let your unconscious mind out for a wander. Seek out hidden meanings and insights.

Surreal (2): It's possible you are experiencing intense feelings about something and need to sort through them, to help make more sense of a situation.

Surreal (3): Your life might be in transition right now, and you are feeling a bit untethered. Perhaps you need to trust your instincts more.

Surreal (4): You could be suppressing your creativity and need to express yourself more often and more clearly. What are you ignoring about yourself?

Surreal (5): You might be feeling bored with routine and need to escape into something more exciting, vibrant, or even strange. Let your imagination soar!

Surreal (6): Consider also if the strange images of these dreams have any specific meanings to you (using this dictionary), as well as how they make you feel.

T

TABLE

Tables are strong objects with solid foundations, but they have multiple different meanings depending on the dream's context:

Broken table (1): There might be problems in your social unit (your family, friends etc.). Something is off, even broken, and you need to find out what it is.

Broken table (2): Also, you might be feeling unsure and unsteady, fearing that you will not be able to "hold up" under the circumstances. Do you need to talk with someone about it?

Building a table: You are probably working on improving connections with others, realizing that we cannot do things alone, and that it often takes a team.

Buying a table: You might be preparing to bring something new into your home or your life (a child, a pet, etc.). It's a fairly big decision and change.

Clearing a table: You could be in store for some unsettling changes in your life, especially when the familiar is removed.

Eating at a table (1): Prosperity and/or good relations with friends and family might be in store for you, if you are enjoying this dream.

Eating at a table (2): If you are experiencing tensions while eating, you could be experiencing the same problems in waking life, or not enjoying the company of others.

Knocking/banging on a table: This dream often indicates arguments, or even people becoming enemies. Who in your life are you banging on tables about?

Long table: Seeing an overly long table in a dream can represent feelings of disconnection, even isolation, from those around you. You might feelleft behind.

Moving table: A table bizarrely moving or walking on its own might suggest that a problem you have will go away by itself. This might be something about you, or something external.

Overturned table: Something has been (or soon will be) turned upside down in your world. This might be good or bad, depending on your circumstances.

Setting the table: You are putting in the work now so that you can reap the benefits to come later, the "feast" that will follow the preparation.

Short/square table: You are probably an organized person who likes everything in its place. You also will probably befriend those who share these beliefs.

Table: A standard table on its own can also represent your sense of security and your relationships to your friends and family.

Tablecloth (clean): A clean tablecloth often symbolizes generosity and a good home life. You either have these things now or would like to.

Tablecloth (dirty): In contrast, a dirty tablecloth can represent arguments and disappointments, and in some cases, disobedience (from children, toward a boss, etc.).

TASTE

You might taste a variety of things in your dreams, and they will have different meanings according to the taste itself:

Bitter: You might be having trouble "swallowing" something unpleasant in your life right now, whether personal or professional, and/or perhaps you feel guilty about something.

Salty: You might be feeling a renewed sense of energy and enthusiasm, as well as feeling better about yourself in a work or personal project.

Sour: Are you feeling resentful about something right now? Has your relationship with someone or something "soured" recently? Either could explain your sour dream.

Sweet: You are probably pleased with your life. You might also be telling yourself to indulge in a little reward for your hard work.

TEA

Tea and drinking tea in dreams usually refers to feelings of calm and being satisfied with your life. You are not pushing yourself too hard and things are going well.

TEETH FALLING OUT

This is an oddly common dream (sometimes the dreamer watches it happen in a mirror) that has several possible meanings:

Dental problems: There might be a very real explanation. A dream of losing teeth can happen to someone facing dental problems, amplified by their imagination and anxiety.

Health concerns: Even without dental problems, any kind of other health issue can cause this dream, as you might be concerned that your health is weakening or falling away.

Lack of control: Watching teeth fall out can leave you feeling helpless, as if control of the situation is gone. Loss of real-life control might bring on this dream.

Loss: You probably have lost something important: a job, a spouse, a death in the family, or something similar, just as our teeth are important to us.

TESTS

Most people don't like taking tests, and dreaming about them usually amplifies that dislike! Here are some possible meanings for your test dream:

Failing a test: You might not feel ready for something in your life, or you could worry that you will never be good enough or measure up to others.

Taking a test (1): You might be apprehensive about something that is coming up, and fear that you haven't prepared for it or done enough work.

Taking a test (2): You might be wrestling with issues of self-esteem and lack of confidence, and/or be worried about others judging you.

Taking a test (3): It's possible that you have strived for too much, set your sights too high, and now you are worried about the outcome.

Taking a test unprepared: Have you been procrastinating something? Your dream might be an expression of you not having faced the issue head on and dealt with it.

THANKS

Giving thanks in a dream can mean that you are feeling grateful in waking life, or that you are finally accepting some part of yourself.

TIME OF DAY

The time of day will often vary widely in dreams, but each specific time can offer us clues about its meaning:

Midnight: A dream about midnight might indicate that you are avoiding something in your life, and you need to face up to it and accept it.

Dawn: You might be feeling renewed and ready to take on a new phase in your life. The darkness is clearing, as is your understanding of your path.

Morning: As you would expect, mornings can symbolize new beginnings and new opportunities, or a chance to start over. Your chance is at hand!

Noon: A dream about noon can indicate that you are at the midpoint of something important in your life. You might also be able to see it more clearly now, in the full light of day.

Afternoon: You have been preparing and now it is time to put those efforts into action. You probably understand a situation better now and can act accordingly.

Dusk: You might be feeling overwhelmed and defeated, as if all of your plans and hopes are for nothing. Darkness is beginning to overtake you.

Night: You are probably facing setbacks in achieving what you want, and you might be feeling that it is difficult to see the issue with any clarity.

TRAPPED

Being stuck in a trap is likely related to you feeling stuck in some way in your daily life: in a job, a relationship, a family situation, etc.

TREES

Trees often feature in the backgrounds of dreams, but if you find yourself noticing them, they can indicate various things:

Barren trees: You might feel as if you've given too much energy to a project or a person, that you are drained and bare. You need to replenish and step back.

Climbing a tree: You are moving up in life, or want to, and seeking to better yourself. This can be in your career, or in some other situation.

Cutting down a tree: This dream might be telling you that you are wasting time and energy on something that is not worth it. Sexual concerns are also possible.

Dead tree: You might be watching a dream die, or a hope come to an end in your waking life. This dream can also point to fertility problems.

Falling tree: Seeing a falling tree can be an indication that you are feeling out of sorts with a situation. You might need to course-correct.

Sitting by or under a tree: If you dream of yourself sitting under a tree, you might be facing an important decision, whether about a situation or a person.

Trees in general: A tree or a group of trees often symbolizes growth and expansion. You are focusing on your own improvement, or you want or need to.

U

UMBRELLA

You probably feel the need to shield yourself from something or someone, or desire shelter and protection, especially if it isn't raining in the dream.

UNDER

If you are under something, you might not be giving yourself enough credit. If you see objects under something, it might be a message from your unconscious. What are the objects?

UNDERGROUND

Dreaming you are underground could mean your unconscious mind is trying to communicate with you, or possibly that you are trying to escape being noticed.

UNDERWEAR

Dreaming about being in public in only your underwear is another common and strange dream. It can mean a few different things depending on what you feel about it:

Confidence: If you are not concerned by walking around in your underwear, you are often ready to reveal something previously hidden about yourself.

Desire to cover up: If you feel the need to put on clothes, you might think that your privacy has been invaded, and/or that others have lost respect for you.

Shame: If you are embarrassed or ashamed, then you might be trying to hide something: feelings, hidden habits, or behaviors that you don't want others to know about.

UNEMPLOYMENT

This dream likely reflects your current job and your feelings around it. You may fear a lack of job security. Alternately, if the emotions in the dream are not negative, perhaps you desire a break or a change of workplace.

UNICORN

This mythical creature often represents luck and good fortune. It is considered an auspicious omen and signifies that good things have come your way or will.

UPSIDE DOWN

Dreaming of being upside down often represent feelings of disorientation, powerlessness, and a lack of belonging. You may also need to change your perspective on something.

V

VACATION

We all need vacations, and we can sometimes dream about them, whether good or bad:

Bad vacation: You are probably not dealing with the problems in your life as well as you'd like. Even when you try to get away from them, they follow you.

On vacation (1): You probably need a vacation, a break from your work and responsibilities. It might not need be a long trip, simply a change from your routine.

On vacation (2): You might also be proud of what you've accomplished and are feeling like you deserve a reward for your hard work. Go ahead and do it!

VACUUM

To dream of a vacuum cleaner illustrates a desire to "clean up" your life or problems and take action into your own hands.

VASE

A vase in a dream typically symbolizes beauty and creativity, especially if it is holding a bouquet of flowers.

VEGETABLES

A dream about vegetables might not be the most exciting thing, but it can mean a few things:

Rotten or withered vegetables: This dream can mean that you are sad about something, or possibly losing something; it is wasting away in front of you.

Specific vegetables: You might be seeking nourishment, whether physical or spiritual. The specific vegetable might suggest a needed nutrient in your diet.

VEIL

To dream of seeing or wearing a veil might indicate that you have aspects about yourself that you want to keep hidden, or you suspect someone else does.

VERTICAL LINE

To see a vertical line can indicate that you have spiritual matters on your mind, and/or want to make a deeper connection with your spiritual side.

VERTIGO

Dizziness and spinning are common in dreams, and often speak to feelings of anxiety, confusion, losing control of a situation, and feeling out of place.

VINES

Flourishing vines may mean that your hard work is paying off; you are or will soon reap the fruits of your labor. If the vines are dry and withered, you may be overextending yourself and need rest.

W

WALL

Walls generally keep things in or out, but their deeper meanings depend on the context of the dream:

Blood on a wall: This unsettling dream usually indicates a warning of some kind. You might fear that someone is spreading rumors about you or talking behind your back.

Building a wall: You are probably trying to keep something or someone out. It could be due to trauma, bad memories, or unpleasant experiences. What are you keeping at bay?

Climbing a wall: You could be trying to overcome some obstacle, but you might need to get help from others to ensure your success.

Collapsed wall: Something has broken down and a turning point is at hand, but this could be for good or ill, depending on your situation.

Crack in the wall: Something is fracturing, possibly a relationship with a friend, partner, or relative. This is an early sign, and you need to work to repair or resolve it.

Destroying a wall: You are trying to overcome one or more obstacles in your life, or free yourself from constraints that you no longer want or need.

Hole in a wall: You might need to be careful with someone, because they could be acting against your interests. The hole can represent the vulnerable point.

House without walls: You're likely dealing with a lack of privacy in your life, or meddling, or you might fear that someone can see into your private thoughts.

Jumping over a wall: If you are able to jump over a wall, you probably have the confidence you need to get past an issue in a situation you are dealing with.

Wall (1): Something is blocking you at the moment. It's a barrier to your progress, whether personally or professionally, and you must deal with it.

Wall (2): Alternately, you might be feeling alienated from others, or trapped in your own ways of thinking and being. What do you need to do to remove that wall?

Writing on the wall: Your unconscious mind is likely sending you a message. Can you read the writing? If not, can you relate it to something in your life that you need to hear?

WAR

To dream about war can be an unsettling, even upsetting experience. Her are some possible interpretations:

War (1): You might need to fight for something you believe in, if you are not doing so already. Or perhaps you are being too combative about something.

War (2): You could be facing some kind of internal struggle, being "at war with yourself." This is unpleasant and needs some kind of resolution, a "peace treaty."

War (3): You might also be worried about actual wars/ conflicts in your area or those of friends and loved ones, and this is expressing itself in your dream.

WARMTH

To be warm in a dream usually means that you are content with your life now, feeling at ease, even cozy. You also are positive about the future.

WATER

Water can come in many forms, and it has diverse meanings in dreams, often to do with the unconscious mind:

Boiling water: You might be suppressing emotions such as anger, hurt, resentment, and they are beginning to bubble up and boil over. They need a release, to "blow off steam."

Clear, calm water: You probably have a clarity of mind and are at peace with yourself, at least about some issue in your life.

Dirty water: You mind is cluttered and you might have bad judgement, or you are hanging onto negative thoughts and feelings that should be let go.

Flooding: Something in your life is out of control or unpredictable. It might be threatening to take down other things in your life if you don't regain that control.

Lake: A dream of a lake can suggest a period of upcoming transition or change. Lakes in myth often hold great power, but also the need for caution.

Ocean: This dream can represent the deep unconscious, and its limitless possibilities. What might you be searching for in those unfathomable depths?

Walking on or over water: You possess self-confidence and control of your emotions, but it might also mean that you have to work to keep your feelings under control.

Waterfalls: A waterfall dream can mean a cleansing is happening or is about to. You might have a chance to wash away the old and have a fresh start.

Waves: Small waves can indicate things coming and going in life, while larger waves (like tidal waves) can warn that you are getting overwhelmed, and your emotion.

WEALTH

To dream that you are wealthy indicates that you are happy with your life and accomplishments, and the wealth you have, whether it's financial, friendship, or love.

WHISPERING

Whether you are whispering or you hear whispering, the dream can have different meanings:

Doing the whispering: You can feel as if you are not being heard, that you lack confidence, or that you have some secret you'd prefer to keep hidden.

Hearing whispering (1): You need to pay closer attention to someone or something in your life. There might be a good reason for doing so if they are speaking to you.

Hearing whispering (2): You might worry that others (for example, at work) are talking about you behind their back, and you have some anxiety about it.

WIDOW(ER)

Dreaming you are a widow when you are not in real life might indicate that you are feeling lost and alone, maybe even abandoned.

WINE

To drink wine in a dream usually denotes satisfaction with your life and reasons to be happy and celebrate. Red wine can also indicate sexual feelings and experiences.

WINTER

Dreaming of winter might suggest feeling stuck or fearing ill health. If, on the other hand, you love winter, the dream might represent the joy of the season and taking time to draw inward.

X

X

To see the letter “x” in a dream can indicate something forbidden to you, whether you want it or not. This could be anything from financial to sexual (see also “Letters of the Alphabet”).

X-RAY

You might need to look inside yourself for the answer you seek, or perhaps you need to investigate a situation much more deeply to avoid being deceived.

Y

YARN

Yarn in a dream symbolizes the interconnectedness of your life. You may find yourself pulled in many directions and need to untangle yourself and focus on what's most important to you.

YAWN

To dream that you are yawning might well mean that you are bored in your waking hours, and need something new and more stimulating. Or your energy levels might be low.

YEARBOOK

Seeing a school yearbook in your dream represents nostalgia and a yearning for something from your past. Perhaps you need to revisit an old hobby you've neglected or catch up with a friend you haven't seen in awhile.

YELLING

Yelling is another expressive dream that can have more than one meaning:

Someone else is yelling: You might be ignoring someone or something in your life that needs attention, possibly a matter that you wanted to leave behind.

You are yelling: You probably have pent-up anger about something and need to release it. This dream is allowing for that, but the situation still needs to be addressed.

You yell, but no one hears: You are likely experiencing frustration and are trying to get someone's attention, and/or you feel that you're being ignored in your waking life.

YES

Saying "yes" in a dream can mean that you are open and accepting of something happening in your life, or maybe that you need to allow yourself to be.

YOGA

Doing or seeing others practice yoga in a dream indicates a desire to connect more with your body. You may want to try the activity in your waking life as well.

YOURSELF

Seeing yourself in a dream (in a mirror, a photo, etc.) is often an indication of how you see yourself in waking life. Is it a positive or a negative view?

Z

ZIG-ZAGGING

If you or someone/something else is moving in zig-zags, it might indicate unpredictable actions and behavior, or that you are trying to avoid something.

ZODIAC

Dreaming about a specific sign could be nudging you to explore its qualities. Dreaming about the whole zodiac might indicate something about the dreamer's views on the passage of time. See "Zodiac Signs."

ZODIAC SIGNS

Each sign can mean different things to the dreamer, especially if they are that sign:

Aquarius: Dreaming about Aquarius can signify looking to the future and trying to be prepared for it. You are welcoming to new ideas, or want to be.

Aries: An Aries dream can refer to your sense of leadership and approaching new things with an enthusiastic mentality. It can also mean the need to face issues directly.

Cancer: To dream about the Cancer sign suggests issues about your emotions and a tendency to be guarded. This can be good or bad, depending on the situation.

Capricorn: To dream about Capricorn might indicate your ambition and goals, but it can also suggest worries about not being good enough and feeling inadequate.

Gemini: Gemini dreams often speak to you having the ability to think quickly and sharply, as well as react to any new situation or challenge.

Leo: A Leo dream might be telling you about your authority (or lack thereof), as well as your creativity and/or need to be the focus of attention from others.

Libra: If you dream about Libra, you might need to restore order and balance in your life, or the dream might speak to your preference for harmony.

Pisces: Your dream of Pisces means you might be willing or needing to sacrifice something for some-one else. Or you might need to change something in your life.

Sagittarius: A Sagittarius dream can indicate that you want to break free from some constraint in your life. It also suggests being adventurous and idealistic.

Scorpio: Scorpio dreams might be indicators of some sexual issue (good or bad), or the need to get to the heart of an issue that is confronting you.

Taurus: You could need to cultivate more tenacity and willpower in your life, basically to be more "bullish." It can sometimes indicate an issue with the neck.

Virgo: A Virgo dream might suggest the need for an emotional release, or speak to your need to be perfect in all your activities (not always a desirable trait).

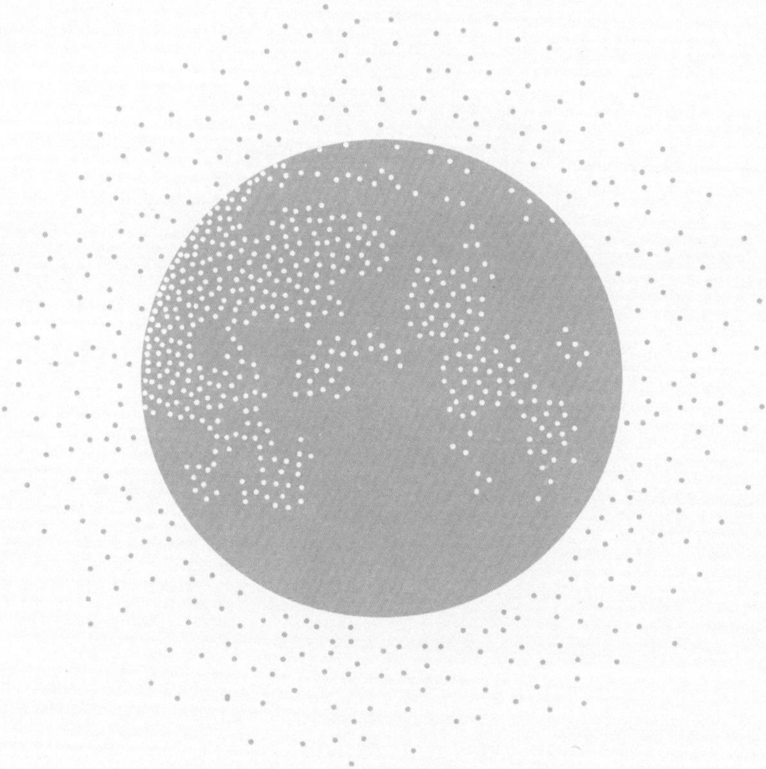

SUGGESTIONS FOR FURTHER READING

There are many books and websites devoted to dreams and their meanings. Often, they will contradict each other, so it's a good idea to read up on several interpretations and make up your own mind about which is the most appropriate meaning for you and your situation.

These resources are a good place to start. The books here will give you a lot of background information on the process of dreaming itself, and theories about what it means for our psyches. There are also a number of websites that have far more entries for dream subjects than a little book like this could possibly contain. Happy searching!

BOOKS

Here are some classic books, as well as newer titles, on all aspects of dreams and dreaming that will offer you detailed background reading and excellent introductions to the fascinating world of dreams:

Sigmund Freud, *The Interpretation of Dreams*

J. Allan Hobson, *A Very Short Introduction to Dreaming*

Robert A. Johnson, *Inner Work: Using Dreams and Active Imagination for Personal Growth*

C.G. Jung, Gerhard Adler (translator), *The Archetypes and the Collective Unconscious*

Josie Malinowski, *The Psychology of Dreaming*

Lisa Marchiano, Deborah Stewart, and Joseph Lee, *Dream Wise: Unlocking the Meaning of Your Dreams*

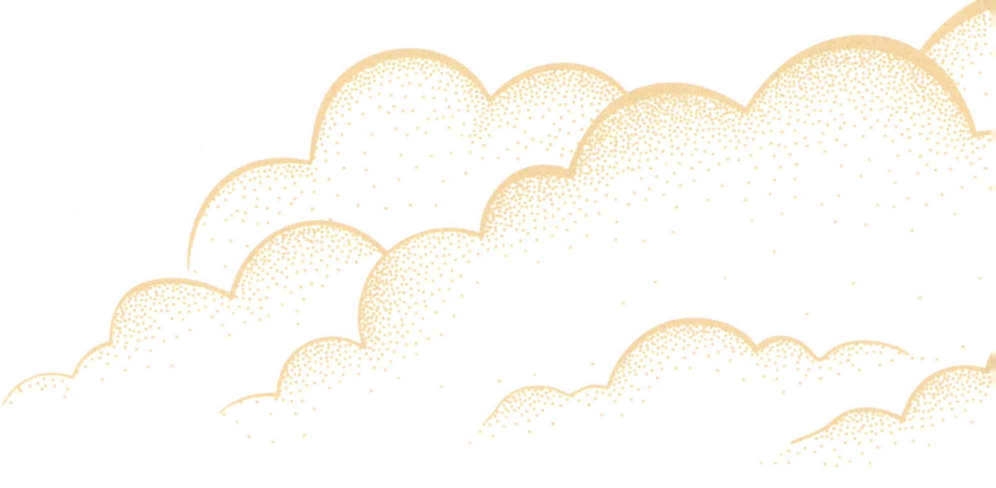

ONLINE RESOURCES

These sites have thousands of entries for all kinds of dreams, and their possible meanings:

www.dreamdictionary.org

www.dreammoods.com

www.sunsigns.com/dreams

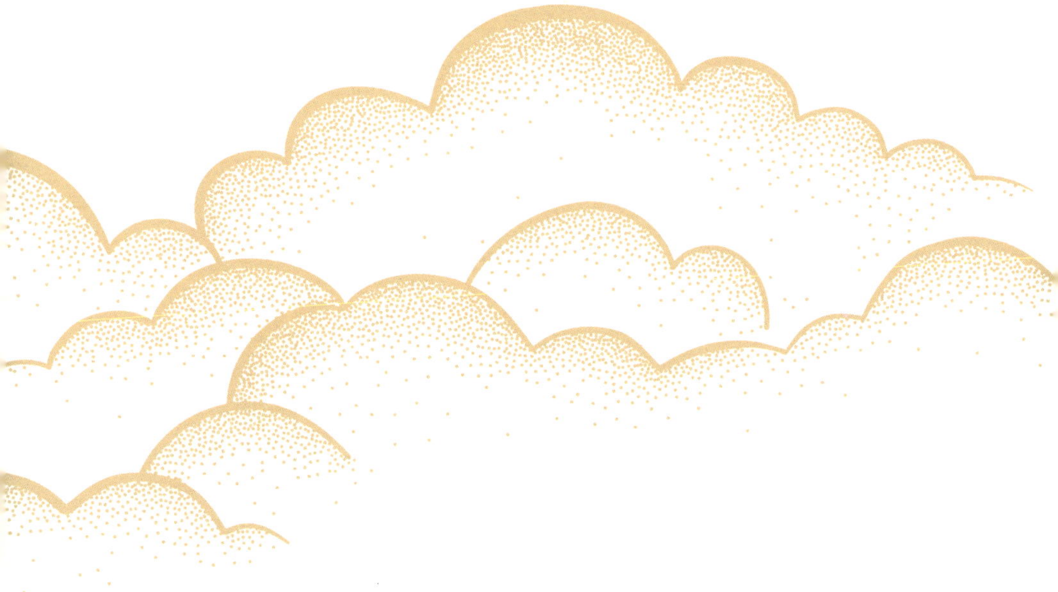

INDEX

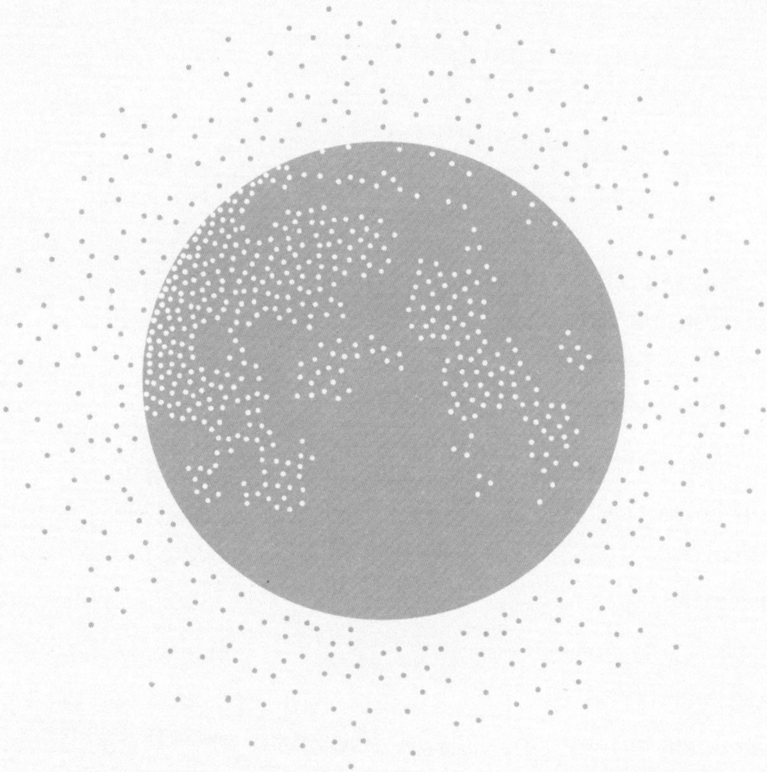

ABOUT THE AUTHOR

Tim Rayborn is an acclaimed and prolific writer of books on many different topics. He has written nearly fifty books about music, the arts, history, the paranormal, mythology, business, and various mind/body/spirit subjects, as well as fantasy and science fiction novels. In addition, he works as a ghost writer, editor, and book coach. Now based in Washington State, he lived in England for seven years and has a PhD in Medieval Studies from the University of Leeds.

He's also an internationally acclaimed musician who plays dozens of unusual instruments and has appeared on over forty recordings. His musical tours and wanderings have taken him across the U.S., all over Europe, and to Canada and Australia.

www.timrayborn.com

MANDALA

An Imprint of MandalaEarth
PO Box 3088
San Rafael, CA 94912
www.MandalaEarth.com

Publisher Raoul Goff
Associate Publisher Roger Shaw
Senior Editor Peter Adrian Behravesh
Assistant Editor Amanda Nelson
Creative Director Ashley Quackenbush
Senior Designer Stephanie Odeh
VP Manufacturing Alix Nicholaeff
Print Production Manager Tiffani Patterson
Strategic Production Planner Lina s Palma-Temena

ISBN: 979-8-88762-158-6

Manufactured in China by Insight Editions

10 9 8 7 6 5 4 3 2 1

ROOTS of PEACE REPLANTED PAPER

Insight Editions, in association with Roots of Peace, will plant two trees for each tree used in the manufacturing of this book. Roots of Peace is an internationally renowned humanitarian organization dedicated to eradicating land mines worldwide and converting war-torn lands into productive farms and wildlife habitats. Roots of Peace will plant two million fruit and nut trees in Afghanistan and provide farmers there with the skills and support necessary for sustainable land use.